MANUAL OF COMMON BEDSIDE SURGICAL PROCEDURES

2ND EDITION

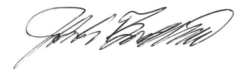

MANUAL OF COMMON BEDSIDE SURGICAL PROCEDURES 2ND EDITION

by the Halsted Residents of the Johns Hopkins Hospital

Editors

Herbert Chen, M.D.
Assistant Chief of Service
Instructor in Surgery
Johns Hopkins Hospital
Johns Hopkins University School of Medicine
Baltimore, Maryland

Christopher J. Sonnenday, M.D.
Senior Resident in General Surgery
Fellow in Surgery
Johns Hopkins Hospital
Johns Hopkins University School of Medicine
Baltimore, Maryland

Consulting Editor

Keith D. Lillemoe, M.D.
Professor of Surgery
Johns Hopkins Hospital
Johns Hopkins University School of Medicine
Baltimore, Maryland

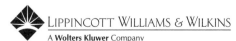

LIPPINCOTT WILLIAMS & WILKINS
A **Wolters Kluwer** Company
Philadelphia · Baltimore · New York · London
Buenos Aires · Hong Kong · Sydney · Tokyo

Editor: Elizabeth Nieginski
Managing Editor: Marette D. Magargle-Smith
Marketing Manager: Aimee Sirmon

The publisher is not responsible (as a matter of product liability, negligence or
otherwise) for any injury resulting from any material contained herein. This
publication contains information relating to general principles of medical care
which should not be construed as specific instructions for individual patients.
Manufacturers' product information and package inserts should be reviewed for
current information, including contraindications, dosages and precautions.

Printed in the Unites States of America

First Edition, 1996

Library of Congress Cataloging-in-Publication Data

Manual of common bedside surgical procedures/by the Halsted residents of the
Johns Hopkins Hospital; editors, Herbert Chen, Christopher J. Sonnenday;
consulting editor, Keith D. Lillemoe. —2nd ed.
    p.;   cm.
  Includes index.
  ISBN 0–683–30792–4
  1. Surgery, Minor—Handbooks, manuals , etc. 2. Clinical medicine—
Handbooks, manuals, etc. I. Title: Common bedside surgical procedures. II. Chen,
Herbert. III. Sonnenday, Christopher J. IV. Lillemoe, Keith D. V. Johns Hopkins
Hospital.
  [DNLM: 1. Surgical Procedures, Minor—methods—Handbooks. WO 39 M294
  2000]
RD111 .M36 2000
617'.024—dc21

                                        99–040830

To purchase additional copies of this book, call our customer service department at
(800) 638-3030 or fax orders to **(301) 824-7390.** International customers should call
(301) 714-2324.

                                 00 01 02 03
                     1 2 3 4 5 6 7 8 9 10

For Harriet, Alex, Elizabeth, Colin, and Sarah
and
For Our Parents,
for their love and inspiration
and
For Christine Martin,
for her everlasting support of the Halsted residents

Previous Editors

First Edition

Herbert Chen, M.D.
Juan E. Sola, M.D.
Keith D. Lillemoe, M.D.

CONTENTS

CHAPTER 3 **CARDIAC PROCEDURES**   **85**

by Sunjay Kaushal, M.D., and Jorge D. Salazar, M.D.

CHAPTER 4 **THORACIC PROCEDURES**   **111**

by Herbert J. Zeh III, M.D.,
and Kevin F. Staveley-O'Carroll, M.D.

CHAPTER 5 **GASTROINTESTINAL PROCEDURES**   **143**

by Robert C. Moesinger, M.D.

CHAPTER 6 NEUROSURGICAL PROCEDURES 179
by Kevin A. Walter, M.D.

CHAPTER 7 UROLOGIC PROCEDURES 205
by Misop Han, M.D.

CHAPTER **PLASTIC AND HAND SURGICAL PROCEDURES**   **237**

by Gregory M. Galdino, M.D.

CHAPTER **ORTHOPEDIC PROCEDURES**   **275**

by Chandrakanth Are, M.D.

CHAPTER 10   NEEDLE BIOPSIES   303

Andrew L. Singer, M.D., and Attila Nakeeb, M.D.

APPENDIX A   LIFE SUPPORT PROTOCOLS   327

by Glen S. Roseborough, M.D.

APPENDIX B   FOCUSED ABDOMINAL SONOGRAPHY FOR TRAUMA (FAST)   345

by Jason Lee Sperry, M.D

APPENDIX C   CONSCIOUS IV SEDATION   349

by Christopher J. Sonnenday, M.D.

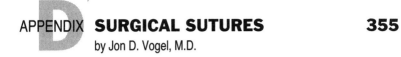

FOREWORD

With the large number of books on the diagnosis and management of patients with surgical diseases, it is almost impossible to find an area or topic not well covered. Among the various publications, there is a great deal of overlap and much repetition. This book, however, *Manual of Common Bedside Surgical Procedures*, has filled a niche where previously there was no satisfactory publication. This second edition amplifies and extends what was initially so successfully presented in the first edition. The procedures and techniques so nicely outlined in this manual are required daily in virtually every hospital in the United States. The responsibility for these procedures in teaching hospitals generally rests with the house staff. Yet in most institutions there is very little in the way of formal instruction on how to perform these procedures, and often the procedures are learned without oversight, on the job, by trial and error. This book provides a detailed overview of how to carry out a variety of procedures, such that any house officer or physician who needs to perform such a procedure is given explicit instruction.

Reading this book does not guarantee that a house officer or physician who has never performed such a procedure before will be able to carry out the task without significant risk of complication. Similarly, a house officer reading a surgical atlas on how to perform a colectomy could not be expected to perform a colectomy for the first time with no supervision without substantial risk of complication. After reading this book, the house officer in many instances will still require oversight and instruction on how to safely carry out the task. This book provides the background information, as well as the anatomical information, that prepares the young physician to perform the procedure. In some instances no further instruction will be needed. In others, formal oversight and instruction by a more experienced physician will be mandatory. The fact that this manual is put together by young house officers who have themselves recently learned how to perform these procedures, and then in turn taught others, makes it a particularly practical and informative publication. Every hospital in the country fortunate enough to have an education program that includes a house staff training program knows the educational benefit of having house officers participating in the care of patients. Over the years all of us on the faculty at Hopkins have learned far more from the surgical house staff than we have been able to teach. They are a stimulus for all of us who are staff surgeons to continue the learning process.

This manual is edited by Dr. Herbert Chen, a Hopkins house officer and one of the original two editors for the first edition, and he is joined by Dr. Christopher J. Sonnenday, also a Hopkins house officer. Dr. Juan E. Sola, who was one of the original editors, has finished his training at Hopkins and currently is on the full-time faculty as a pediatric surgeon at the Miami Children's Hospital. The consulting editor remains Dr. Keith D. Lillemoe, who is the coordinator of our Residency Training Program in Surgery at Hopkins. Of the many important educational activities that our house staff at Hopkins participate in, this is one of the most visible, but only one of many aimed at medical students, residents, and surgical attendings. All eventually result in what we all strive for, improved patient care.

John L. Cameron, M.D.
1999

PREFACE (FIRST EDITION)

As the care of patients continues to become more complex and technologically oriented, there has been an increase in the number of invasive monitoring, diagnostic, and therapeutic procedures performed at the bedside. In many situations, these procedures are performed by surgical house officers on an elective and sometimes emergent basis. Although surgical residents will acquire the skills to perform the procedures by experience and "hands-on" instruction, a manual detailing and carefully illustrating the many diverse procedures would be beneficial. Currently, techniques for performing some bedside procedures can be found in subspecialty texts, but there is no convenient manual solely devoted to bedside procedures including techniques from a variety of medical fields.

Manual of Common Bedside Surgical Procedures is a useful, transportable, and fully illustrated text that attempts to accomplish this goal. The chapters on airway management and arterial/venous access are crucial to all house officers. Cardiothoracic, abdominal, and needle biopsy procedure chapters are especially useful to surgical residents. The chapters covering neurosurgical, urologic, plastic surgical, and orthopedic procedures can serve as quick references for intermittently performed procedures. Junior residents and medical students will find this entire manual to be a useful tool while first learning these procedures.

Manual of Common Bedside Surgical Procedures is edited by two current and one former Halsted resident. The chapters are written by the house officers of the Johns Hopkins Hospital, including Halsted surgical residents. The technical aspects of and the systematic approach to performing bedside procedures have been passed down from one resident to another over the years. By having residents as authors, the individuals actually performing these techniques are imparting important, first-hand knowledge targeted to other residents who will be performing these tasks. It was the dedication of these residents that made this book possible.

This text in no way aims to replace the "hands-on" instruction and experience needed to be accumulated by an individual prior to performing bedside procedures. No one should attempt a technique if they do not have adequate experience or supervision. Finally, the techniques described in this manual reflect the experience of the chapter authors, and may need to be be modified depending on each individual resident and each patient.

H. C.
J. E. S.
K. D. L.

PREFACE (SECOND EDITION)

We are extremely pleased to provide a second edition of *the Manual of Common Bedside Surgical Procedures* by the Halsted residents of the Johns Hopkins Hospital. We have received positive feedback from numerous residents throughout the country who have used the first edition. Furthermore, the success of the manual overseas has been impressive. Currently, *the Manual of Common Bedside Surgical Procedures* is translated into nine foreign languages: French, Spanish, Japanese, Chinese, Turkish, Persian, Russian, Indonesian, and Polish.

Despite all of this, we have tried to improve the manual in this latest edition. This updated version has several new additions. The chapters on airway management, arterial/venous access, thoracic procedures, urologic procedures, plastic surgery and hand procedures, and needle biopsies include new or revised techniques. Furthermore, we have added to the Appendix sections on focused abdominal sonography for trauma (FAST) and surgical sutures. While making these modifications, we have maintained many of the features that our readers liked about the first edition: detailed illustrations; a wide variety of surgical procedures; portable size; and easy-to-read, step-by-step instructions.

This second edition would not have been possible without the foundation laid by the editors of the first edition. Since the last edition, Dr. Juan Sola has finished his training in general and pediatric surgery at Johns Hopkins. Dr. Keith Lillemoe remains at Johns Hopkins as Professor of Surgery, but has taken a consulting editor role in the second edition. The contributions of these two individuals cannot be understated, and we are grateful for their past and continuing role in the education of the Halsted surgical residents.

H.C.
C.J.S.

ACKNOWLEDGMENTS

Manual of Common Bedside Surgical Procedures represents the dedication and hard work of the contributors as well as the current and former Halsted residents. We are especially grateful to those who made contributions to the first edition: Stephen A. Barnes, M.D.; Elizabeth A. Davis, M.D.; Jay H. Epstein, M.D.; Cora Lee Foster, M.D.; Peter J. Gruber, M.D., Ph.D.; Paul P. Lin, M.D.; Jennifer M. Lindsey, M.D.; Peter Mattei, M.D.; Thomas J. Polascik, M.D.; Prakash Sampath, M.D.; C. Max Schmidt, M.D., M.B.A.; Juan E. Sola, M.D.; and Bernadette H. Wang, M.D.

We were very fortunate to have the talents of our illustrator, Kimberly Battista, for a second time. The success of the first edition was greatly due to her superb illustrations. Her latest drawings in this new edition continue in her line of excellence.

Many others have also helped us along the way. They include Robert Udelsman, M.D.; H. Kim Lyerly, M.D.; Michael A. Choti, M.D.; Herbert J. Zeh III, M.D.; and Robert A. Montgomery, M.D., Ph.D.

We again would like to thank John L. Cameron, M.D., the Chairman of the Department of Surgery and Surgeon-in-Chief of the Johns Hopkins Hospital. Dr. Cameron has followed in the great tradition of Halsted and Blalock in creating a residency that stands alone in clinical and academic excellence combined with an unsurpassed history and tradition. In addition, we are grateful to Keith D. Lillemoe, M.D., the Vice-Chairman of the Department of Surgery and Professor of Surgery, for his role as senior consulting editor and advisor to us and to the majority of surgical residents at Johns Hopkins.

Lastly, our efforts would not be possible without the support of our families. We sincerely appreciate their understanding, care, and devotion.

CONTRIBUTORS

All contributors are from the Johns Hopkins Hospital and the Johns Hopkins University School of Medicine, Baltimore, Maryland.

Chandrakanth Are, M.D.
Senior Resident in General Surgery, Fellow in Surgery

Herbert Chen, M.D.
Assistant Chief of Service and Instructor, Department of Surgery

Gregory M. Galdino, M.D.
Senior Resident in General Surgery, Fellow in Surgery

Christine G. Cattaneo, M.D.
Fellow in Anesthesia and Critical Care Medicine

Misop Han, M.D.
Senior Resident in Urologic Surgery

Sunjay Kaushal, M.D.
Senior Resident in General Surgery, Fellow in Surgery

Catherine Marcucci, M.D.
Assistant Professor, Department of Anesthesia and Critical Care Medicine

Robert C. Moesinger, M.D.
Assistant Chief of Service and Instructor, Department of Surgery

Attila Nakeeb, M.D.
Assistant Chief of Service and Instructor, Department of Surgery

Glen S. Roseborough, M.D.
Fellow in Vascular Surgery

Jorge D. Salazar, M.D.
Chief Resident in General Surgery, Fellow in Surgery

Andrew L. Singer, M.D.
Senior Resident in General Surgery, Fellow in Surgery

Christopher J. Sonnenday, M.D.
Senior Resident in General Surgery, Fellow in Surgery

Julie Ann Sosa, M.D.
Senior Resident in General Surgery, Fellow in Surgery

Jason Lee Sperry, M.D,
Senior Resident in General Surgery, Fellow in Surgery

Kevin F. Staveley-O'Carroll, M.D.
Assistant Chief of Service and Instructor, Department of Surgery

Jon D. Vogel, M.D.
Senior Resident in General Surgery, Fellow in Surgery

Kevin A. Walter, M.D.
Senior Resident in Neurosurgery

Herbert J. Zeh III, M.D.
Senior Resident in General Surgery, Fellow in Surgery

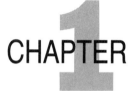

CHAPTER

AIRWAY MANAGEMENT

Authors: Christine G. Cattaneo, M.D., Catherine Marcucci, M.D., and Herbert Chen, M.D.

AIRWAY MANAGEMENT

The establishment and management of a patent airway is the first principle of resuscitation and life support; it is an essential skill for all house officers. This skill is predicated on a thorough knowledge of airway anatomy.

A. MANUAL AIRWAY MANEUVERS—HEAD TILT AND JAW THRUST

1. Indications:
   a. Initial management of a compromised airway
   b. Stimulus to respiratory drive in the sedated patient
   c. Relief of mild anatomic airway obstruction (snoring, etc.)

2. Contraindications (to Head Tilt):
   a. Suspected cervical spine injury
   b. Down's syndrome (due to incomplete C1–C2 ossification and cervical vertebral subluxation)
   c. Previous cervical fusion
   d. Known cervical spine pathology (ankylosing spondylitis, arthritis, rheumatoid arthritis)

3. Anesthesia:
   None

4. Equipment:
   None

5. Positioning:
   Supine

6. Technique—Head Tilt:
   a. If any of the contraindications above apply, use jaw thrust only.

b. Tilt head back on atlanto-occipital (C1) joint while keeping mouth closed; head remains in neutral position.
c. Lift chin to facilitate elevation and anterior movement of hyoid bone away from pharyngeal wall (see Figure 1.1).

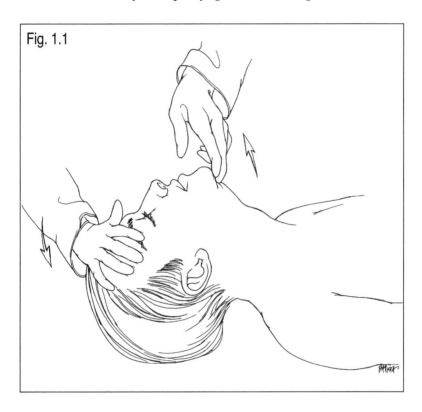

Fig. 1.1

7. Technique—Jaw Thrust:

a. Open mouth slightly; gently depress mentum with thumbs.
b. Grip mandibular rami with fingers, and lift the mandibular teeth over and in front of maxillary teeth (see Figure 1.2).
c. A two-handed technique works best because the elasticity of the mandibular joint capsule and masseter muscle will pull the mandible back into the joint if the grip is relaxed.

8. Complications and Management:

In children under age 5 years, the cervical spine can bow upward with manual maneuvers. Such maneuvers can worsen the obstruction by pushing the posterior pharyngeal wall upward

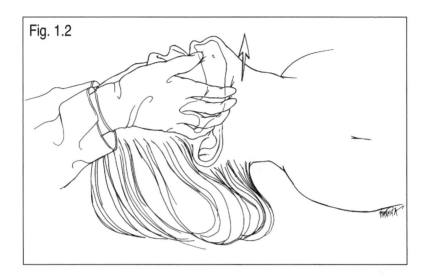

Fig. 1.2

against the tongue and epiglottis. In children, the airway is best maintained by leaving the head in a neutral position.

B. ORAL AIRWAY DEVICES

1. Indications:
   a. Complete or partial obstructed upper airway
   b. Bite block in the unconscious or intubated patient
   c. Adjunct for oropharyngeal suctioning

2. Contraindications:
   a. Dental or mandibular fracture
   b. History or acute episode of reactive airway disease

3. Anesthesia:
   10% topical lidocaine spray to suppress gag response

4. Equipment:
   a. Plastic or elastomeric flanged oral airway
   b. Tongue depressor
   c. Suction apparatus

5. Positioning:
   Supine or lateral

6. Technique:
    a. Open mouth; place tongue blade at base of tongue; draw the tongue anteriorly to lift it off of the pharynx.
    b. Place airway in the mouth with the concave side facing the mentum so that the distal end is approximating but not touching the posterior wall of the oropharynx; flange and 1–2 cm of the shaft of the airway should protrude above the incisors.
    c. Perform the jaw thrust maneuver to lift the tongue off of the pharyngeal wall.
    d. Tap the airway down the last 2 cm so that the curve lies beyond the base of the tongue.
    e. Alternatively, the airway may be inserted with concave side facing the palate. Insert in mouth until tip is past the uvula (no tongue blade required); rotate 180° to sweep under the tongue from the side. This method of twisting the oral airway in the mouth is not recommended if the patient has poor dentition or oral trauma, because the teeth may be further dislodged or the bleeding increased.

7. Complications and Management:
    a. Exacerbation of reactive airway disease
        • Maintain airway with maneuver described in Section A.
    b. Retching or vomiting
        • Turn the head to the side and suction.
    c. Increased airway obstruction if not properly placed
        • Remove the device and re-insert if needed.

C. NASAL AIRWAY DEVICES

1. Indications:
    a. Upper airway obstruction in awake or semicomatose patients
    b. Dental or oropharyngeal trauma
    c. Inadequate airway patency after placement of oral airway device

2. Contraindications:
    a. Nasal occlusion
    b. Nasal fractures or basal skull fractures
    c. Deviated septum
    d. Coagulopathy

    e. Cerebrospinal fluid (CSF) rhinorrhea

    f. Previous transsphenoidal hypophysectomy

    g. Previous posterior pharyngeal flap for repair of craniofacial defects

    h. Pregnancy (due to vascular engorgement of the nasal passages after the first trimester)

3. Anesthesia:

    a. Gauge patency of nares by visual inspection (relative size, presence of bleeding or polyps) or by exhalation test.

      • Have the patient exhale through nose onto small hand-held mirror or shiny bevel of laryngoscope blade.

      • Relative size of condensation indicates which naris is more patent.

    b. Mix a slurry (generally 10 mg phenylephrine in 10 ml of 2% lidocaine jelly) to provide topical anesthesia and vasoconstriction of the nasal airway.

    c. Swab lidocaine jelly mixture just inside external edge of naris until local anesthesia occurs.

    d. Gently place successive swabs deeper into naris until three swabs can comfortably be placed simultaneously to the level of the posterior nasal wall.

    e. If three cotton swabs can be accommodated, a 7.5-mm airway will usually pass.

    f. If swabs are not available, the lidocaine mixture may be syringed directly into the nose.

4. Equipment:

    a. Cotton swabs

    b. Graduated sizes of nasal airways (generally 6.0 through 8.0 mm)

    c. 2% lidocaine jelly

    d. Phenylephrine

    e. Suction apparatus

5. Positioning:

    Supine, lateral, or sitting

6. Technique:

    a. Pass the airway gently into the nose with the concave side facing the hard palate.

b. The airway follows a path through the nose that is parallel to the palate and under the inferior turbinate.

c. If resistance is met in the posterior pharynx, bend the tube 60°–90° with gentle pressure to proceed down the pharynx; it also may be helpful to rotate the airway 90° counterclockwise and rotate it back to the original position as it makes the bend down the pharynx.

d. If the airway will not pass with moderate pressure, a narrower airway should be used.

e. If the airway still does not advance, withdraw it 2 cm and pass a small suction catheter through it, then push the airway forward, using the catheter as a guide.

f. If still unsuccessful, the naris can be re-dilated or the other naris can be prepped and used.

7. Complications and Management:

a. Epistaxis
- Pack anterior superficial bleeders per Section H.
- Consult otolaryngology service for posterior bleeding.

b. Submucosal tunneling
- Remove device.
- Patient may require plastic surgical repair.

D. BAG–MASK VENTILATION

1. Indications:

a. Spontaneous ventilation absent or inadequate
b. Preliminary preoxygenation when intubation is planned
c. Short-term oxygenation when ventilation is temporarily compromised

2. Contraindications:

a. Hiatal hernia
b. Suspicion of active or passive regurgitation
c. Need to avoid head and neck manipulation
d. Tracheoesophageal fistula
e. Tracheal fracture or laceration
f. Facial fractures or trauma
g. Severe disruption of dermal surface
h. Full stomach (relative)

3. Anesthesia:

None

4. Equipment:

a. Fitted face mask with collar
b. Respiratory or resuscitator (Ambu) bag
c. O_2 supply
d. Suction apparatus

5. Positioning:

Supine, head in anatomic "sniffing" position

6. Technique:

a. Place an oral (Section B) or nasal (Section C) airway.
b. Hold the mask in the left hand; the thumb and index finger grip the mask around the collar with the body of the mask fitting into the left palm.
c. Place the narrow end of the mask on the bridge of the nose, avoiding pressure on the eyes.
d. Lower the body of the mask to the face so the chin section of the mask rests on the alveolar ridge.
e. Seal the contact areas with the midsection of the face by pulling the mandible up into the mask with the curled fingers of the left hand and tilting the mask slightly to the right (see Figure 1.3).
f. Deliver intermittent breaths with the right hand on the bag.
g. In a spontaneously breathing patient, time the delivered breaths to coincide with the patient's inhalations.
h. In the tachypneic patient, alternate the assisted breaths with spontaneous respirations.
i. Buccal gauze sponges can be placed in the cheeks of an edentulous patient to improve fit to the face. Care must be taken not to increase airway obstruction; if this occurs, remove sponges immediately.
j. In very difficult mask airways, the mask may be fitted to the face with both hands as an assistant delivers breaths (see Figure 1.4).

7. Complications and Management:

a. Acute gastric distension
   • Requires placement of a nasogastric tube to decompress the stomach
b. Vomiting

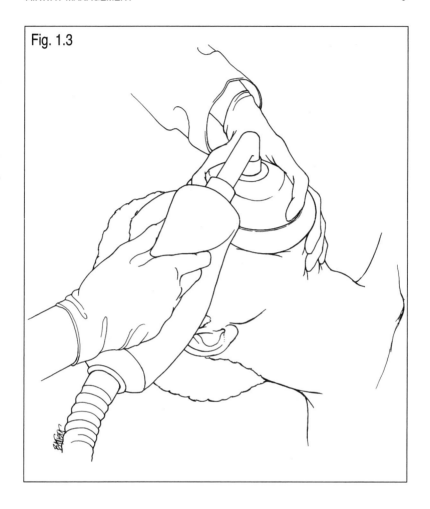

Fig. 1.3

E. TRACHEAL INTUBATION—ORAL AND NASAL

Nasal intubation is generally performed in the awake, spontaneously breathing patient when there is an advantage to avoiding laryngoscopy.

1. Indications:
   a. PO_2 decreased from age-appropriate level
   b. PCO_2 increased from baseline
   c. Change in mental status
   d. In the adult patient, respiratory rate fewer than 7 breaths per minute or greater than 40 breaths per minute
   e. Inability to protect airway

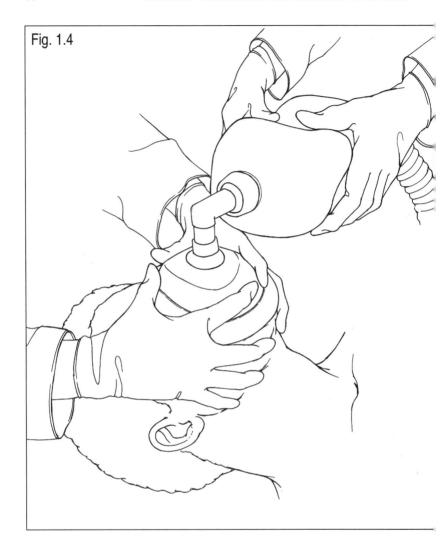

Fig. 1.4

f. Anticipated cardiovascular or respiratory collapse (sepsis, severe burn, etc.)
g. Anticipated bronchoscopic evaluation

2. Contraindications:
   a. Oral intubation
      • Tracheal fracture or disruption
   b. Nasal intubation
      • Pregnancy (due to vascular engorgement of the nasal passages after the first trimester)

- Coagulopathy
- Nasal occlusion
- Nasal fracture
- Deviated septum
- CSF rhinorrhea
- Previous transsphenoidal hypophysectomy
- Previous posterior pharyngeal flap for repair of craniofacial defects

3. Anesthesia:

Frequently, an induction agent and a neuromuscular blocking agent are administered to facilitate intubation; a sedative is commonly given afterward to lessen agitation in the awake, intubated patient.

- a. Induction agents
  - Thiopental (4–6 mg/kg)
  - Etomidate (0.3 mg/kg)
  - Ketamine (1–3 mg/kg)
- b. Neuromuscular blocking agents
  - Succinylcholine (1.0 mg/kg)
  - Vecuronium (0.3 mg/kg for rapid sequence induction)
- c. Sedatives
  - Diazepam (0.03–0.1 mg/kg)
  - Midazolam (0.05–0.15 mg/kg)
- d. Resuscitation drugs should be available at the bedside: atropine, phenylephrine, ephedrine, and epinephrine.
- e. Use topical lidocaine spray to anesthetize the airway when intubation of awake patient is planned.

4. Equipment:

- a. Rigid laryngoscope blade and handle (see Figure 1.5)
- b. Ambu bag and mask
- c. O_2
- d. Suction apparatus
- e. Styletted endotracheal tubes (ETT) in varying sizes (usually 6.0 through 8.0 mm for adults)

5. Positioning:

- a. Supine with head in sniffing position if patient is already horizontal or unconscious, or if oral intubation is planned
- b. May remain sitting for blind nasal intubation if the patient cannot tolerate lying flat

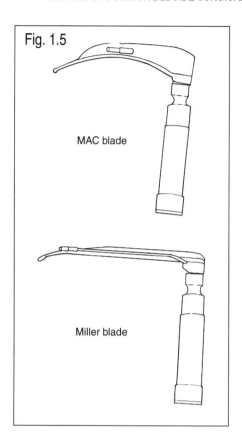

Fig. 1.5

MAC blade

Miller blade

6. Technique—Oral Intubation:

a. Check the ETT cuff for leaks by inflating and deflating the balloon with 10 ml of air.

b. Check the blade and handle to ensure that the light is functioning.

c. Preoxygenate with mask ventilation; have assistant apply cricoid pressure (see Figure 1.6).

d. Remove oral airway.

e. Grasp laryngoscope blade and handle in left hand.

f. Instruct the awake patient to open the mouth as widely as possible. In the unconscious patient, place the thumb and second fingers of the right hand on the right upper and lower molars and open the mouth with a scissor-like motion, subluxating the jaw out of the temporomandibular joint.

g. Gently place the laryngoscope blade in the right side of the mouth, taking care to avoid damaging the teeth (see Figure 1.7).

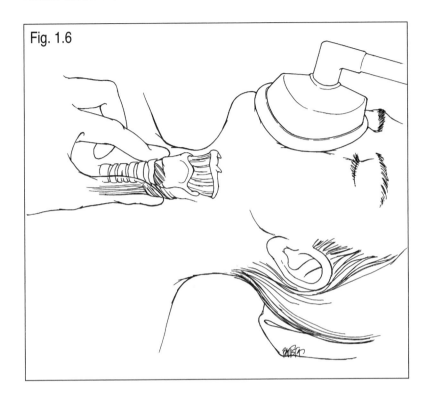

Fig. 1.6

h. Move the tongue to one side of the oral cavity while advancing the blade toward the glottic opening (see Figure 1.8).

i. Position the end of the blade under the epiglottis or in the vallecula, depending on the type of blade used (see Figures 1.9 and 1.10).

j. With the left wrist in an unbroken position, firmly lift the laryngoscope handle toward an imaginary point above the patient's left foot to expose the vocal cords. It is extremely important to avoid cocking the left wrist backward and levering the blade on the teeth.

k. Pass the styletted tube with the cuff deflated into the right side of the mouth and through the vocal cords; have an assistant remove the stylet as the cuff passes through the vocal cords to avoid damage to the trachea.

l. Place the ETT so that the cuff is just distal to the cords (cannot be seen between or above the cords); inflate the balloon with 5–10 ml of air and hold the tube firmly in place at the lips.

m. Place the portable end-tidal CO_2 monitor in the breathing circuit between the tube adaptor and the ventilator bag; gently give several breaths. Watch the chest for expansion. Check a

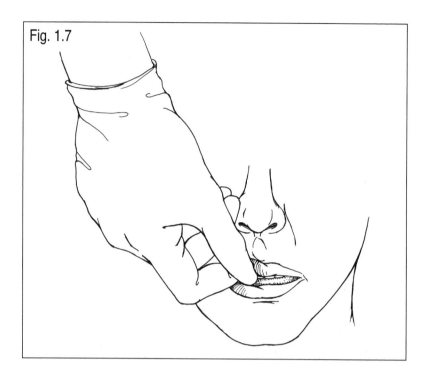

Fig. 1.7

     minimum of six breaths for measurement of CO_2 on the CO_2 monitor; this is to ensure that the CO_2 returned to the breathing circuit has a pulmonary source and is not insufflated air from the stomach. Listen for bilateral breath sounds over the chest and for an absence of sounds over the gastric area.

n. If all clinical signs point to intubation of the trachea, the assistant may release the cricoid cartilage when instructed to do so.

o. Tape the tube securely. Carefully place an oral airway, or in an awake patient, place a bite block to avoid obstruction of the tube by biting.

p. Obtain a chest radiograph to check ETT placement.

q. If more than one intubation attempt is necessary, the patient should have a mask airway re-established between attempts.

r. If the esophagus is intubated inadvertently (in a case in which the vocal cords are difficult to visualize), it may be helpful to leave the ETT in place as a marker to avoid repeated esophageal placements.

s. Inadequate mouth-opening is a common mistake and can make laryngoscopy unnecessarily difficult as well as greatly increase the risk of dental damage.

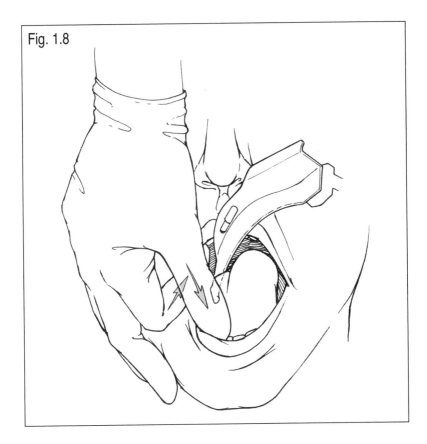

Fig. 1.8

t. Exposure and visualization of the vocal cords is usually eas-
   ier with a Miller blade; however, passing the ETT can be
   more difficult because the view of the cords is sometimes obstructed by the tube as it passes through the oral cavity and
   supraglottis. Retraction of the right cheek and placing the
   ETT from the lateral side of the right molars can be helpful.

7. Technique—Nasal Intubation:
   a. Check the ETT cuff for leaks by inflating and deflating the
      balloon with 10 ml of air.
   b. Check the function of the laryngoscope light source.
   c. Nasal intubation is generally done in the awake, sponta-
      neously breathing patient when there is an advantage to
      avoiding laryngoscopy (cervical neck fracture, etc.).
   d. Prepare the naris as for a nasal airway.
   e. Use nasal airways to dilate the naris; generally the ETT used

Fig. 1.9

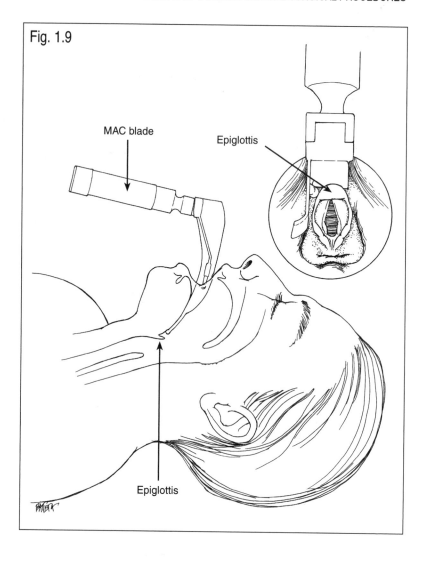

will be one size smaller than the largest nasal airway that can be comfortably placed.

f. Coat the end and cuff of an unstyletted tube with viscous lidocaine jelly; if warm saline is available, the tube may first be soaked for 3 minutes and then preformed with a gentle curve about 3 cm from the end to facilitate passage under the epiglottis.

g. Place gently in the nose; advance the tube using the technique described for placing the nasal airway; gently extend the neck if the tube is difficult to pass.

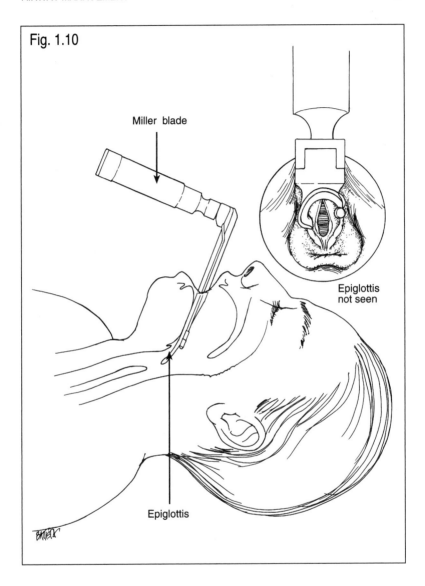

Fig. 1.10

Miller blade

Epiglottis not seen

Epiglottis

h. Watch the tube for signs of fogging as the tube approaches the vocal cords; quality of the voice may also change (see Figure 1.11).

i. Ask the patient to breathe deeply, and gently advance the tube through the cords while they are open during inspiration; the patient should immediately lose phonation.

j. Inflate the cuff, verify position, and secure as for an oral ETT. An oral airway is not necessary.

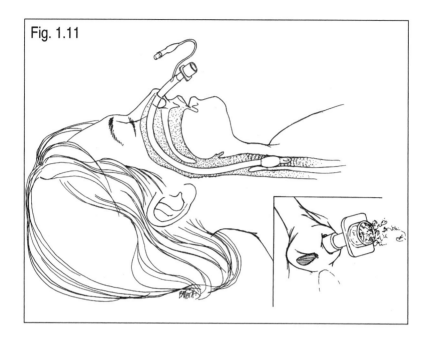

Fig. 1.11

8. Complications and Management:
   a. Minor airway damage
      • Inspect for lacerations to tongue, lips, and gums to ensure that any bleeding has stopped.
      • Repair lacerations if necessary.
   b. Dental damage
      • Immediate retrieval of any dislodged teeth is mandatory.
      • Consult the dental or ENT service for further management.
   c. Esophageal intubation
      • Decompress the stomach.
   d. Major airway trauma
      • Obtain chest radiograph.
      • Perform emergent cricothyroidotomy if needed (see Section H).
      • Consult the ENT service immediately.

F. LARYNGEAL MASK AIRWAY

1. Indications:
   a. Airway is completely or partially obstructed
   b. Alternative to ventilation with bag–mask or ETT
   c. Mask ventilation or endotracheal intubation is difficult

2. Contraindications:
   a. Dental or mandibular fracture
   b. History or acute episode of reactive airway disease
   c. Pharyngeal abscess or obstruction
   d. Full stomach (e.g., trauma, pregnancy, obesity)
   e. Need for mechanical positive pressure ventilation
   f. Foreign body in airway

3. Anesthesia:

   The laryngeal mask airway (LMA) can be used in the heavily sedated, spontaneously breathing patient or during general anesthesia with or without neuromuscular blockade.
   a. Heavy sedation without neuromuscular blockade
      • Midazolam (0.5–1.5 mg/kg)
      • Propofol (25–100 µg/kg/min)
   b. Induction agents
      • Thiopental (4–6 mg/kg)
      • Propofol (1–2.5 mg/kg)
      • Etomidate (0.3 mg/kg)
      • Ketamine (1–3 mg/kg)
   c. Neuromuscular blocking agents
      • Succinylcholine (1 mg/kg)
      • Rocuronium (0.6 mg/kg)
   d. Resuscitation drugs should be readily available—atropine, phenylephrine, epinephrine.

4. Equipment:
   a. LMA, appropriately sized
   b. 20-ml syringe
   c. Gauze bite-block
   d. Suction apparatus
   e. Tape
   f. O_2 source
   g. Ambu bag/mask

5. Positioning:

   Supine

6. Technique:
   a. Check the LMA cuff for leaks by inflating and deflating LMA with 20–30 ml of air.

b. Fully deflate and smooth out wrinkles in cuff.
c. Lubricate the back of the cuff.
d. With the right hand, open mouth with thumb and second finger on lower and upper incisors, respectively, using a scissor-like motion.
e. Grasp the LMA in left hand, and slide it over the tongue (with lubricated back of LMA against the palate) into the hypopharynx until resistance is met (see Figure 1.12).

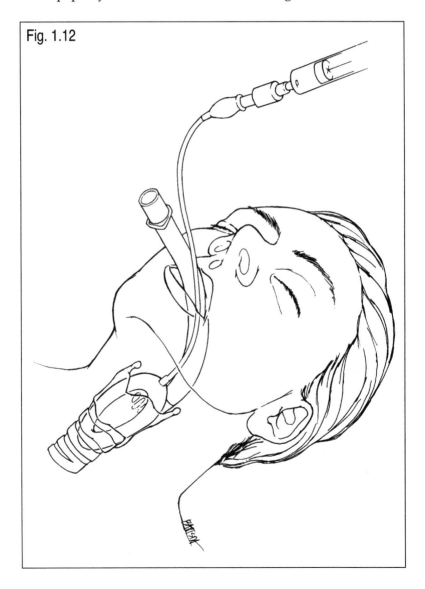

Fig. 1.12

    f. Inflate the cuff with 20–30 ml of air.

    g. Examine the patient for bilateral breath sounds, using either spontaneous or mechanical ventilation.

    h. When assured of correct placement, secure LMA to face with tape.

    i. Insert gauze bite-block between upper and lower teeth to prevent obstruction of the tube by biting.

7. Complications and Management:

    a. Dental damage
- Immediately retrieve any dislodged teeth.
- Consult dental service for further management.

    b. Regurgitation of gastric contents
- If emesis occurs, suction oropharynx, remove LMA, and place ETT as described.

G. LIGHT WAND TRACHEAL INTUBATION

1. Indications:

    a. Alternative to direct laryngoscopy

    b. Difficult conventional intubation

2. Contraindications:

    a. Known anatomical abnormalities in oropharynx or upper airway

    b. Epiglottitis

    c. Foreign body in airway

    d. Upper airway trauma

    e. Patients with limited neck extension/cervical spine disease

    f. Morbid obesity

3. Anesthesia:

Endotracheal intubation with a light wand requires general anesthesia with neuromuscular blockade (as described in oral and nasal tracheal intubation).

4. Equipment:

    a. Light wand

    b. ETT, appropriately sized

    c. 10-ml syringe

   d. Water-soluble lubricant
   e. Suction apparatus
   f. O_2 source
   g. Ambu bag/mask
   h. Tape

5. Positioning:

   a. Supine
   b. Head and neck in neutral position (in contrast to anatomical "sniffing" position for direct laryngoscopy)

6. Technique:

   a. Test the ETT cuff with 10 ml of air, then deflate.
   b. Lubricate the length of the light wand with a water-soluble lubricant.
   c. Place the light wand inside the ETT, and align the light wand length markings with those of the ETT; this will place the light source at the end of the ETT without any protrusion beyond the tip of the ETT. Secure ETT position by locking light wand adaptor around ETT connector (see Figure 1.13).
   d. Bend the ETT–light wand at the designated location on the proximal end of the light wand into a 90° angle.
   e. Standing behind the patient's head, use the nondominant hand to grasp the patient's mandible (place the thumb inside the patient's mouth to secure the tongue against the mandible) and lift away from the posterior pharynx.
   f. With dominant hand, slide the concave angle of the ETT–light wand over the midline of the tongue into the posterior pharynx.
   g. Gently rock the ETT–light wand back and forth along the midline until a discreet glow appears on the neck slightly superior to the sternal notch (indicating correct placement of the light source into the glottis).
   h. Stabilize the ETT–light wand in position, retract the stiff internal stylet of the light wand, and advance the ETT–light wand into the trachea.
   i. Release the ETT from the light wand by unlocking the adaptor and removing the light wand while firmly holding the ETT in position.
   j. Inflate the ETT cuff, listen for bilateral breath sounds, and check for end-tidal Co_2.
   k. When assured of correct placement, secure the ETT to the

Fig. 1.13

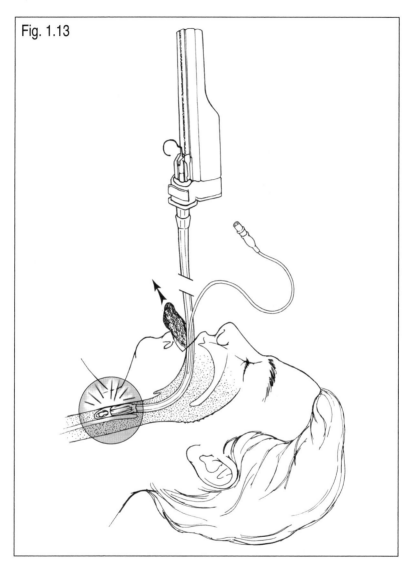

face with tape. Carefully place an oral airway or bite block in an awake or nonparalyzed patient to avoid obstruction of the ETT by biting.
   l. Obtain chest radiograph to confirm ETT placement.

7. Complications and Management:

   a. Dental damage
   As described above

b. Disconnection of light source from light wand
  • Ensure correct ETT placement.
  • Consult otolaryngology service for removal of foreign body.
c. Subluxation of cricoarytenoid cartilage—rarely occurs if stiff stylet is correctly withdrawn before ETT–light wand is advanced into trachea.
  • As above, ensure correct ETT placement.
  • Consult ENT service.

H. SURGICAL CRICOTHYROIDOTOMY

1. Indications:

a. Extensive orofacial trauma preventing laryngoscopy
b. Upper airway obstruction secondary to edema, hemorrhage, or foreign body
c. Unsuccessful endotracheal intubation and need for emergent airway

2. Contraindications:

Children under age 12 years. Needle cricothyroidotomy is preferred to avoid damage to cricoid cartilage (see next section).

3. Anesthesia:

None

4. Equipment:

a. Scalpel blade and handle
b. Tracheal spreader
c. Tracheostomy tube or ETT (6F–8F)
d. Sterile prep solution, gloves, and towels
e. Ambu bag and oxygen
f. 3-O silk ties
g. Hemostats

5. Positioning:

Supine, with neck in neutral position. In trauma patients, a cervical spine injury must be assumed until radiological and clinical examination have excluded this diagnosis.

6. Technique:

a. Sterile prep and drape the neck.
b. Make a longitudinal 3- to 4-cm incision in the midline of the neck from the thyroid cartilage down past the cricothyroid membrane (see Figure 1.14)

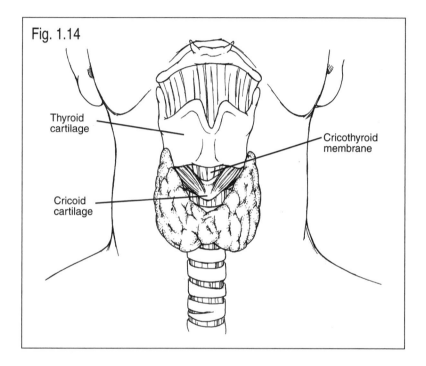

Fig. 1.14

Thyroid cartilage

Cricothyroid membrane

Cricoid cartilage

c. Palpate the cricothyroid membrane below the thyroid cartilage in the midline. Stabilize the thyroid cartilage with the non-dominant hand and make a transverse incision approximately 2 cm through the cricothyroid membrane with a scalpel(see Figure 1.15).
d. Insert tracheal spreader into the trachea and gently spread. If a tracheal spreader is not available, insert the handle of the scalpel into the trachea and turn the scalpel 90° to enlarge the opening in the cricothyroid membrane.
e. Insert the tracheostomy tube and remove tracheal spreader.
f. Inflate cuff with 5 ml of air, attach Ambu bag, and ventilate patient with 100% oxygen.
g. Auscultate the chest to confirm equal and clear breath sounds bilaterally.

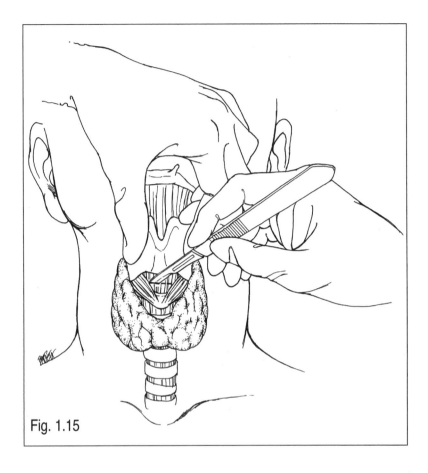

Fig. 1.15

   h. Control superficial bleeding either with direct pressure or
      with hemostats and 3-O silk ligatures if necessary.

7. Complications and Management:
   a. Bleeding
      • Usually superficial and self-limited
      • Control with direct pressure or sutures.
   b. Esophageal injury
      • Can occur if scalpel penetrates the posterior
        trachea.
      • Keep incision superficial, stopping once cricothyroid
        membrane is incised.
      • If esophageal injury is suspected, obtain surgical
        consultation.

I. NEEDLE CRICOTHYROIDOTOMY

An acceptable alternative to surgical cricothyroidotomy and the preferred technique in children. However, needle cricothyroidotomy can only provide adequate ventilation for only 30–45 minutes.

1. Indications:
   a. Extensive orofacial trauma preventing laryngoscopy
   b. Upper airway obstruction secondary to edema, hemorrhage, or foreign body
   c. Unsuccessful endotracheal intubation
   d. Preferred method of obtaining emergent airway in children under age 12 years

2. Contraindications:
   None

3. Anesthesia:
   None

4. Equipment:
   a. 12- to 14-gauge angiographic catheters
   b. 3.0-mm pediatric ETT adaptor
   c. Y connector
   d. Oxygen supply with flow meter
   e. Oxygen tubing
   f. 5-ml syringe
   g. Sterile prep solution and gloves

5. Positioning:
   Supine, with neck in neutral position. In trauma patients a cervical spine injury must be assumed until radiological and clinical examination have excluded this diagnosis.

6. Technique:
   a. Sterile prep and drape the neck (see Figure 1.16).
   b. Palpate the cricothyroid membrane below the thyroid cartilage in the midline.
   c. Attach a 5-ml syringe to a 12- to 14-gauge angiographic

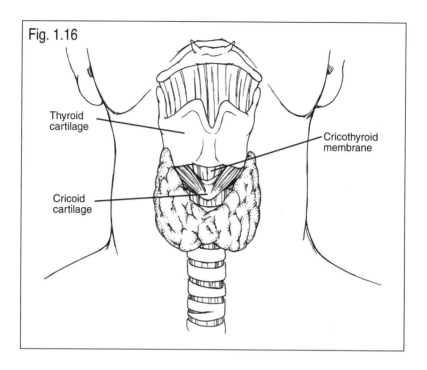

Fig. 1.16

Thyroid cartilage

Cricothyroid membrane

Cricoid cartilage

catheter, and puncture the skin in the midline over the cricothyroid membrane. Direct catheter inferiorly at 45° to the skin (see Figure 1.17).

d. Advance the catheter while aspirating. Stop once air is aspirated, which confirms position within the tracheal lumen.

e. Advance the catheter over the needle down the distal trachea, and withdraw the needle.

f. Attach a 3.0-mm pediatric ETT adaptor to hub of catheter.

g. Attach a Y connector to oxygen tubing and to pediatric ETT adaptor.

h. Maintain oxygen flow at 15 L/min.

i. Provide ventilation by intermittently placing thumb over open end of Y connector for 1 second and off for 4 seconds.

7. Complications and Management:

a. Bleeding
   • Usually superficial and self-limited
   • Control with direct pressure or sutures.

b. Esophageal injury
   • Can occur if angiographic catheter penetrates the posterior trachea.

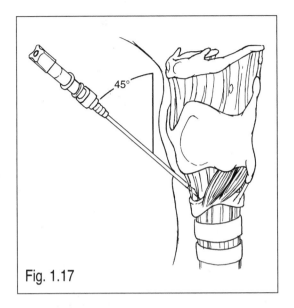

Fig. 1.17

- Stop advancing catheter once air is aspirated.
- If esophageal injury is suspected, obtain surgical consultation.

J. NASAL PACKS

1. Indications:

   Persistent nasal bleeding despite simple first aid measures.

2. Contraindications:

   None

3. Anesthesia:
   a. Cocaine solution (2.5%–10%) or 2% lidocaine
   b. 1:1000 epinephrine

4. Equipment:
   a. Headlight
   b. Forceps
   c. Suction catheter
   d. Silver nitrate sticks

e. Lubricated ribbon gauze (0.5–1 inch)
f. Foley catheter
g. Syringe, 10 ml

5. Positioning:

Sitting

6. Technique:

a. Assess patient's general condition to determine effect of blood loss already sustained. Any patient who appears to be in shock should have a baseline hemoglobin, platelet count, prothrombin time, partial thromboplastin time, and cross-matching of blood while resuscitation with crystalloid fluid is underway. In contrast, if the patient is hypertensive, reassurance and antihypertensives should be administered to control the BP.

b. Stable patients should then be assessed sitting in a well-illuminated area where suction is available.

c. Initially have patient pinch nostrils between finger and thumb continuously for 10 minutes. Apply ice pack to bridge of nose.

d. If bleeding persists, remove blood clots from nose either with forceps or suction catheter.

e. Insert two cotton swabs soaked with 10% cocaine or 2% lidocaine and 1:1000 epinephrine into bleeding nostril. This will anesthetize the nasal mucosa and vasoconstrict blood vessels.

f. Carefully inspect the nasal mucosa, searching for a bleeding point.

g. If bleeding has stopped, the patient should be observed for 1–2 hours to ensure that no further treatment is required.

h. If bleeding persists from a visible site, it should be chemically cauterized. After anesthetizing the area again with 10% cocaine solution, touch the bleeding point with a silver nitrate stick until hemostasis is achieved.

i. If bleeding continues without an identifiable source, nasal packing will be required.

j. Insert one end of the lubricated ribbon gauze (0.5–1 inch) along the floor of the nostril as far posteriorly as possible. Introduce folds lengthwise from floor to roof of the nasal cavity until it is firmly filled. Generally, 100 cm of ribbon gauze can be inserted without difficulty (see Figure 1.18).

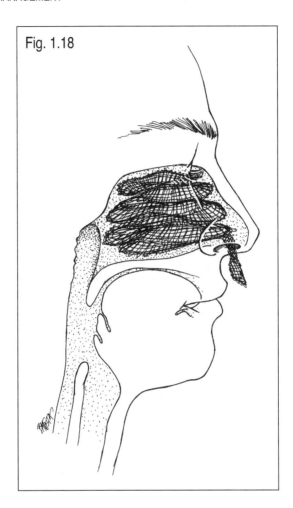

Fig. 1.18

k. Pack may be left in place for 2–3 days with prophylactic oral antibiotics and ENT follow-up to remove pack.
l. If bleeding persists, a posterior nasal pack will be required. Remove anterior nasal pack and insert a Foley catheter along the floor of the nostril until the tip of the catheter reaches the nasopharynx (see Figure 1.19).
m. Inflate balloon with 10 ml of air, and withdraw catheter until balloon blocks posterior choana.
n. Tape catheter firmly to nostril to prevent balloon from falling into oropharynx.
o. Patient with posterior nasal packs will require hospitalization and prophylactic antibiotics.

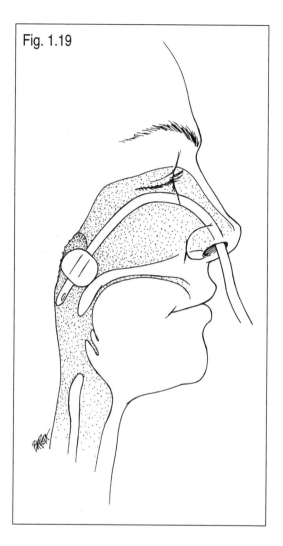

Fig. 1.19

7. Complications and Management:

   a. Persistent or recurrent bleeding
   - If anterior and posterior packs fail, surgical ligation of the maxillary and anterior ethmoidal arteries will be required.
   - Obtain ENT consultation.
   b. Infection
   - Can occur with obstruction of the eustachian tube
   - Prophylactic antibiotics should be administered to patients with nasal packs, along with instructions to seek medical care immediately if fever or discharge occur.

- If infection is suspected, remove pack immediately.
c. Hypoxemia
    - May occur, because nasal packs compromise respiration
    - Elderly patients or those with respiratory problems should be admitted for observation.

CHAPTER 2

ARTERIAL AND VENOUS ACCESS

Authors: Julie Ann Sosa, M.D. and Herbert Chen, M.D.

VENOUS AND ARTERIAL ACCESS

I. CENTRAL VENOUS ACCESS

Central venous catheters are frequently used in the intensive care unit (ICU) and operating room for monitoring and for venous access. Although this procedure is routine for most surgical house officers, central line insertion should be approached with caution and adequate preparation. Patient positioning is crucial to success. Informed consent should be obtained prior to performing elective access procedures, and bleeding parameters (i.e., hematocrit, platelet count, and PT/PTT ratios) should be optimized.

A. SUBCLAVIAN VENOUS ACCESS—TWO APPROACHES

1. Indications:
   a. Central venous pressure (CVP) monitoring
   b. Total parenteral nutrition (TPN)
   c. Long-term infusion of drugs
   d. Inotropic agents
   e. Poor peripheral access

2. Contraindications:
   a. Venous thrombosis
   b. Coagulopathy (PT or PTT >1.5 × control)
   c. Untreated sepsis
   d. For the standard (infraclavicular) approach: need for hemo-

dialysis access, because there is an association with subclavian vein stenosis

3. Anesthesia:

   1% lidocaine

4. Equipment:
   a. Sterile prep solution
   b. Mask, sterile gown, gloves, towels, dressings
   c. 22- and 25-gauge needles
   d. 5-ml syringes (two)
   e. Shoulder roll towel
   f. Appropriate catheters and dilator
   g. Intravenous (IV) tubing and flush
   h. 18-gauge insertion needle (5–8 cm long)
   i. 0.035 J-shaped wire
   j. Scalpel
   k. 2-0 silk suture

5. Positioning:

   Supine, in Trendelenburg. Place a towel roll between the scapulas underneath the thoracic vertebrae as shown. Allow the patient's shoulders to fall down and back (or have an assistant apply gentle traction to the ipsilateral arm), and have the patient's head turned away from the side of the line placement (see Figure 2.1).

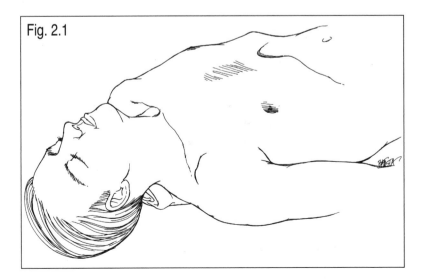

Fig. 2.1

6. Technique—Standard (Infraclavicular) Approach:

a. In a sterile fashion, dress with mask and gown and prep and drape the patient's left or right subclavian area. It is often useful to prep the ipsilateral neck into the sterile field in case it is necessary to attempt an internal jugular vein approach.

b. Place an index finger at the sternal notch and the thumb at the intersection of the clavicle and first rib (see Figure 2.2).

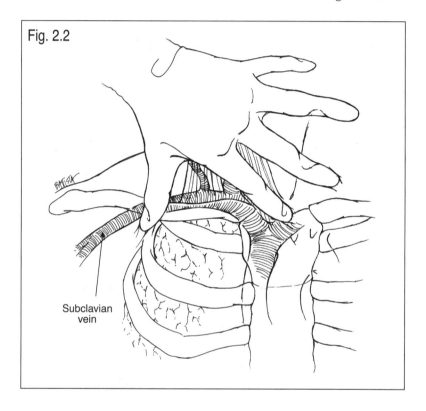

Fig. 2.2

Subclavian
vein

Administer 1% lidocaine with a 25-gauge needle into the skin and subcutaneous area 2 cm lateral to your thumb and 0.5 cm caudal to the clavicle. Use a 22-gauge needle to anesthetize the periosteum of the clavicle 2–3 cm lateral to the first rib intersection. Always aspirate before injecting.

c. Using the 18-gauge insertion needle with a 5-ml syringe, puncture the skin that is lateral to your thumb and 0.5 cm caudal to clavicle. While aspirating, slowly advance the needle underneath the clavicle toward your index finger at the sternal notch. The needle must be horizontal (parallel to the

floor) at all times to avoid pneumothorax, and the bevel
should be facing up or toward the patient's feet to encourage
the guidewire to advance toward the heart rather than into
the neck. The needle may be depressed with your thumb to
get underneath the clavicle (see Figure 2.3).

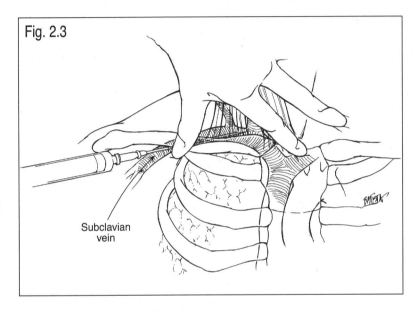

Fig. 2.3

Subclavian
vein

d. If there is no venous blood return after advancing 5 cm,
   slowly withdraw needle while aspirating (the needle might
   have punctured both vessel walls). After completely withdrawing needle, redirect it, aiming 1 cm above sternal notch.
   If there is still no venous blood return, reanesthetize the skin
   1 cm lateral puncture site rather than previous site and reattempt access. If still unsuccessful, consider moving to the
   contralateral side after obtaining a portable chest radiograph
   (CXR) to rule out pneumothorax.
e. If air or arterial blood is encountered, stop immediately and
   see complications section.
f. If venous access is obtained with good flow, remove syringe
   while keeping a finger over the needle to prevent air embolism.
g. Introduce the J wire, with the tip aimed toward the heart,
   through the needle while maintaining the needle in the
   same location (Seldinger technique). The wire must pass
   with minimal resistance. Note that if an inferior vena cava

(IVC) filter is known to be in place, use the non-J end of the wire to avoid snaring the filter in case the wire is advanced through the heart and into the IVC.

h. If resistance is met, remove the wire, check needle placement by withdrawing blood with a syringe, and if good flow is obtained, introduce the wire again while turning the patient's head to the ipsilateral side (to close the angle that would allow the wire to ascend the ipsilateral jugular vein).

i. Once the wire is passed, remove the needle while keeping control of the wire at all times.

j. Enlarge the puncture site with a sterile scalpel.

k. While keeping control of the wire, introduce the dilator over the wire 3–4 cm to dilate the subcutaneous tissues (see Figure 2.4). Advancing the dilator the entire length can lacerate the subclavian vein and is not recommended.

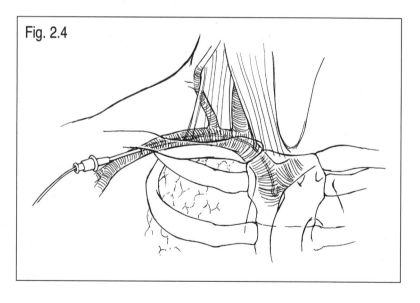

Fig. 2.4

l. Remove the dilator, and introduce the central venous catheter over the wire to the length of 15 cm on the right and 18 cm on the left (see Figure 2.5).

m. Remove the wire, aspirate blood from all ports to confirm venous placement, and then flush with sterile saline. Suture the catheter to the skin, and apply sterile dressing.

n. Run IV fluids at 20 ml/hr and order a portable CXR to confirm placement in superior vena cava (SVC) and rule out pneumothorax.

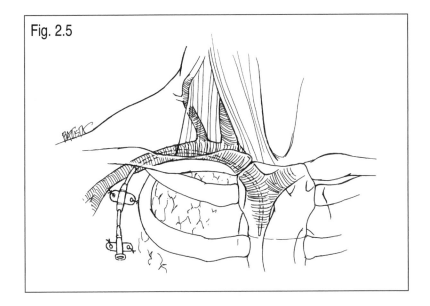

Fig. 2.5

7. Technique—Supraclavicular Approach:
   a. In a sterile fashion, dress with mask and gown and prep and
      drape the patient's left or right subclavian area. It is often
      useful to also prep the ipsilateral neck into the sterile field in
      case it is necessary to attempt an internal jugular vein ap-
      proach.
   b. Select an insertion site 1 cm medial and superior to the mid-
      point of the clavicle (preferably the right, to avoid injury to
      the thoracic duct). Administer 1% lidocaine with a 25-gauge
      needle into the skin and subcutaneous tissue.
   c. Direct an 18-gauge introducer needle attached to a syringe
      toward the sternoclavicular joint 20° cephalad to the trans-
      verse plane of the clavicle and 20° anterior to the coronal
      plane of the patient. Maintain gentle aspiration until the vein
      is entered, usually at a depth of 2 cm. The vein puncture site
      is posterior to the clavicular head of the sternocleidomastoid
      muscle and medial to the subclavian artery pulsation. The
      vein is entered at the confluence of the subclavian and inter-
      nal jugular veins (see Figure 2.6).
   d. If air or arterial blood is encountered, stop immediately and
      see complications section.
   e. If venous access is obtained with good flow, remove the sy-
      ringe while keeping a finger over the needle to prevent air
      embolism and introduce the J wire, following the same

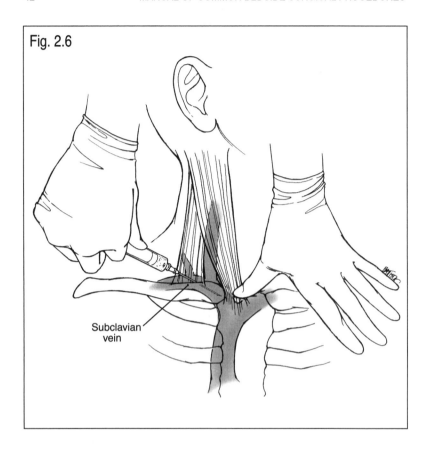

Fig. 2.6

Subclavian
vein

Seldinger technique described above for the infraclavicular
approach.

8. Complications and Management:

a. Arterial puncture
  - Withdraw needle immediately, and apply manual pressure
    for 5 minutes.
  - Monitor hemodynamics and breath sounds for
    hemothorax.

b. Air embolus
  - Attempt to withdraw air by aspirating through catheter.
  - If hemodynamically unstable (cardiac arrest), initiate
    Advanced Cardiac Life Support (ACLS) protocol and
    thoracic surgery consultation.
  - If stable, position patient in left lateral decubitus and
    Trendelenburg position to trap air in right ventricle.

CXR in this position can show significant air and be used for follow up.
- Air will eventually dissolve.

c. Pneumothorax
- If a tension pneumothorax is suspected, decompress with 16-gauge angiographic catheter in the second intercostal space, midclavicular line.
- If < 10%, 100% oxygen and serial CXRs
- If > 10%, tube thoracostomy

d. Malpositioning
- Into right atrium (RA) or right ventricle (RV), against wall of vein—withdraw or advance as needed to place in SVC.
- Into other subclavian vein—stable position, no adjustment needed
- Into jugular or mammary vein—reintroduce J wire, remove catheter, thread long 18-gauge angiographic catheter and confirm placement in vein by aspiration of blood. The J wire can now be redirected into SVC by maximizing positioning (pull caudally on arm, and turn the head and neck ipsilaterally to close internal jugular vein angle).

e. Dysrhythmias
- Atrial or ventricular dysrhythmias are associated with wires and catheters in the RA or RV and usually resolve after withdrawing the catheter into the SVC.
- Persistent dysrhythmias may need medical management.

B. INTERNAL JUGULAR VENOUS ACCESS—TWO APPROACHES

1. Indications:
   a. CVP monitoring
   b. TPN
   c. Long-term infusion of drugs
   d. Inotropic agents
   e. Hemodialysis
   f. Poor peripheral access

2. Contraindications:
   a. Previous ipsilateral neck surgery
   b. Untreated sepsis
   c. Venous thrombosis

3. Anesthesia:

1% lidocaine

4. Equipment:

a. Sterile prep solution
b. Mask, sterile gown, gloves, and towels
c. 22- and 25-gauge needles
d. 5-ml syringes (two)
e. Appropriate catheters and dilator
f. IV tubing and flush
g. 18-gauge insertion needle (5–8 cm long)
h. 0.035 J wire, sterile dressings
i. Scalpel
j. 2-0 silk suture

5. Positioning:

Supine, in Trendelenburg. Turn the patient's head 45°
contralaterally to expose the neck (see Figure 2.7).

6. Technique—Central Approach:

a. In a sterile fashion, dress with mask and gown. Identify the
apex of the triangle formed by the heads of the sternocleidomastoid muscles (SCM), and prep and drape this area. Also
locate the external jugular vein and the carotid artery (see
Figure 2.8). It is often useful to prep the ipsilateral clavicle
artery into the sterile field in case it is necessary to attempt
the subclavian approach.
b. Administer anesthetic with 25-gauge needle into skin and
subcutaneous tissue at the apex of the triangle. Always withdraw before injecting because the vein can be very superficial.
c. Palpate the carotid pulse and apply gentle traction medially
with the other hand.
d. Insert the 22-gauge finder needle with a syringe at the apex
of the triangle 45°–60° to the skin and advance it slowly toward the ipsilateral nipple while aspirating.
e. If there is no venous blood return after 3 cm, slowly withdraw needle while aspirating. If still no return, redirect the
needle through the same puncture site aiming 1–3 cm more
laterally and then, if unsuccessful, 1 cm medially. Watch the
carotid artery. If there is still no blood return, reassess land-

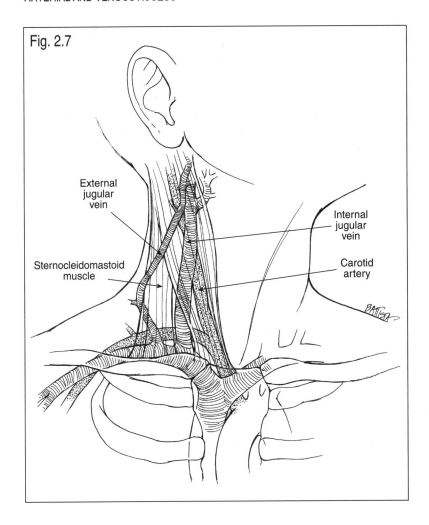

Fig. 2.7

External jugular vein

Internal jugular vein

Sternocleidomastoid muscle

Carotid artery

marks and consider posterior approach if unable to obtain access after three attempts.

f. If air or arterial blood is encountered, stop immediately and see complications section.

g. If good venous return, memorize the site and angle of entry of the finder needle and then remove the needle. Apply digital pressure to minimize bleeding. Alternatively, the needle may be left in place as a guide.

h. Insert the 18-gauge needle, following the same angle as the finder needle (see Figure 2.9).

i. If venous access is obtained with good flow, remove syringe while keeping a finger over the needle to prevent air embolism.

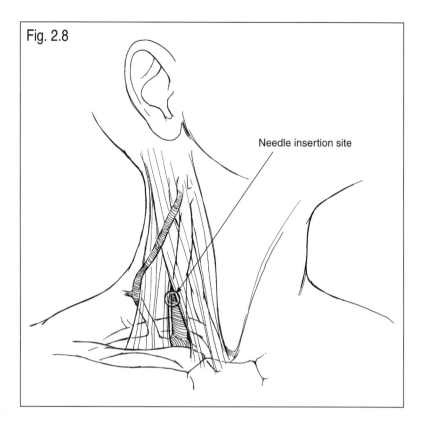

Fig. 2.8

Needle insertion site

j. Introduce the J wire, with the tip aimed toward the heart (medially), through the needle while maintaining the needle in the same location (Seldinger technique). The wire must pass with minimal resistance.

k. If resistance is met, remove the wire, check needle placement by withdrawing blood with a syringe, and reintroduce wire if good blood return.

l. Once the wire is passed, remove the needle while keeping control of the wire at all times.

m. Enlarge the puncture site with a sterile scalpel.

n. Introduce the venous catheter over the wire while maintaining a constant hold on the wire to the length of about 9 cm on the right and 12 cm on the left.

o. Remove the wire, aspirate blood from all ports to confirm venous placement, and then flush with sterile saline. Suture the catheter to the skin and apply sterile dressing.

p. Run IV fluids at 20 ml/hr and order a portable CXR to confirm placement in SVC and rule out pneumothorax.

Fig. 2.9

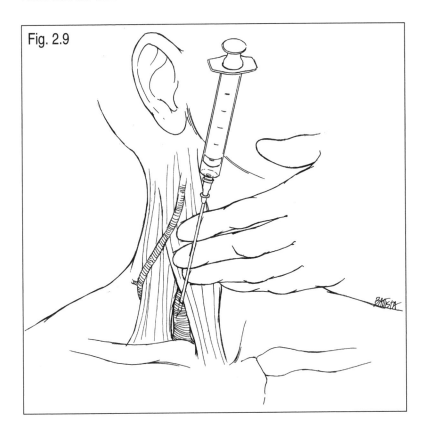

7. Technique—Posterior Approach:

  a. In a sterile fashion, dress with mask and gown. Identify the
     lateral border of the SCM where the external jugular vein
     crosses over it. It is about 4–5 cm above the clavicle (see Fig-
     ure 2.10). It is often useful to prep the ipsilateral clavicle into
     the sterile field in case it is necessary to attempt the subcla-
     vian approach.

  b. Administer anesthetic with a 25-gauge needle into skin and
     subcutaneous tissue 0.5 cm superior to the intersection of the
     SCM and external jugular vein. Always withdraw before in-
     jecting because the vein can be very superficial.

  c. Insert the 22-gauge finder needle with a syringe at point A
     and advance slowly anteriorly and inferiorly toward the
     sternal notch while aspirating (see Figure 2.11).

  d. If there is no venous blood return after 3 cm, slowly with-
     draw needle while aspirating. If there is still no return, redi-
     rect the needle through the same puncture site aiming

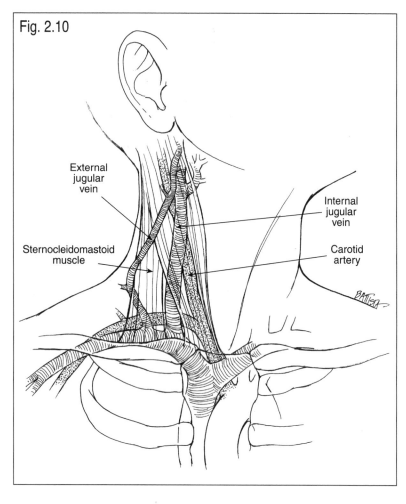

Fig. 2.10

External
jugular
vein

Internal
jugular
vein

Sternocleidomastoid
muscle

Carotid
artery

slightly ipsilateral to the sternal notch. If there is still no
blood return, reassess landmarks and consider attempting
the contralateral side after three attempts. CXR must be obtained to rule out pneumothorax before changing sides.
  e. If air or arterial blood is encountered, stop immediately and
     see complications section.
  f. If good venous return, memorize the site and angle of entry
     of the finder needle and then remove the needle. Apply digi-
     tal pressure to minimize bleeding. Alternatively, the needle
     may be left in place as a guide.
  g. Insert the 18-gauge needle, following the same angle as the
     finder needle. If venous access is obtained with good flow,
     remove syringe while keeping a finger over the needle to

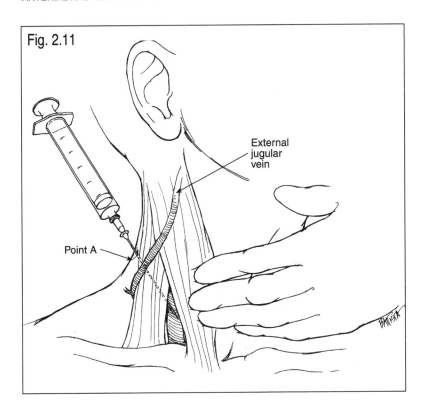

Fig. 2.11

External jugular vein

Point A

prevent air embolism and introduce the J wire, following the same Seldinger technique described above for the central approach.

8. Complications and Management:
   a. Carotid puncture
      • Withdraw needle immediately and apply manual pressure.
      • If cannulation occurred and manual pressure is not successful, surgical intervention may be needed.
   b. Air embolus
      • Attempt to withdraw air by aspirating through catheter.
      • If hemodynamically unstable (arrest), initiate ACLS protocol and thoracic surgery consultation.
      • If stable, position patient in left lateral decubitus and Trendelenburg position to trap air in right ventricle. CXR in this position can show significant air and be used for follow up.
      • Air will eventually dissolve.

   c. Pneumothorax
      • If a tension pneumothorax is suspected, decompress with
        16-gauge angiographic catheter in the second intercostal
        space, midclavicular line.
      • If < 10%, 100% oxygen and serial CXRs
      • If > 10%, tube thoracostomy
   d. Malpositioning
      • Into RA or RV, against wall of vein—withdraw or advance
        as needed to place in SVC.
      • Into subclavian vein—stable position, no adjustment
        needed.
      • Into jugular or mammary vein—re-introduce J wire,
        remove catheter, thread long 18-gauge IV catheter and
        confirm placement in vein by aspiration of blood. The J
        wire can now be redirected into SVC by maximizing
        positioning (pull caudally on arm and turn the head and
        neck ipsilaterally to close internal jugular vein angle).
   e. Horner's syndrome
      • Puncture of the carotid sheath can result in a temporary
        Horner's syndrome that usually resolves.
   f. Dysrhythmias
      • Atrial or ventricular dysrhythmias are associated with
        wires and catheters in the RA or RV and usually resolve
        after withdrawing the object into the SVC.
      • Persistent dysrhythmias may need medical
        management.

C. FEMORAL VENOUS ACCESS

1. Indications:
   a. Emergent central access
   b. Hemodialysis
   c. Unable to obtain subclavian or internal jugular venous ac-
      cess for CVP or inotropic agents

2. Contraindications:
   a. Prior groin surgery (relative)
   b. Patient must maintain bed rest while the catheter is in place

3. Anesthesia:
   1% lidocaine

4. Equipment:
   a. Sterile prep solution
   b. Mask, sterile gown, gloves, and towels
   c. 25-gauge needle
   d. 5-ml syringes (two)
   e. Appropriate catheters and dilator
   f. IV tubing and flush
   g. 18-gauge insertion needle (5 cm long)
   h. 0.035 J wire, sterile dressings
   i. Safety razor
   j. Scalpel
   k. 2-0 silk suture

5. Positioning:
   Supine

6. Technique:
   a. In a sterile fashion, dress with mask and gown. Shave, prep, and drape left or right groin area.
   b. Palpate the femoral pulse at the midpoint along an imaginary line between the anterior superior iliac spine and the symphysis pubis. The femoral vein runs parallel and immediately medial to the artery (see Figure 2.12).
   c. Administer anesthetic with 25-gauge needle into the skin and subcutaneous tissue 1 cm caudally and laterally to the palpated pulse.
   d. Retracting the artery laterally with your finger, use the 18-gauge insertion needle with a 5-ml syringe to puncture the skin. Advance the needle while aspirating cranially at a 45° angle to the skin, parallel to the pulse. There is less risk with being medial to the vein rather than lateral to it (see Figures 2.13 and 2.14).
   e. If there is no venous blood return after 5 cm, slowly withdraw needle while aspirating. If still no return, redirect the needle through the same puncture site, aiming in a cranial and more lateral direction 1–2 cm closer to the artery.
   f. If still no blood return, reassess landmarks and attempt access 0.5 cm medial to the femoral pulse.
   g. If arterial blood is encountered, withdraw needle and hold manual pressure according to the complications section.
   h. If venous access is obtained with good flow, remove syringe while keeping a finger over the needle to prevent air embolism.

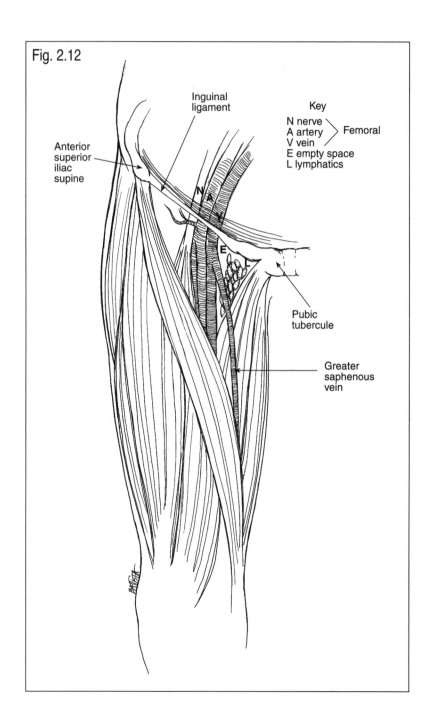

Fig. 2.12

Inguinal
ligament

Key

N nerve
A artery   Femoral
V vein
E empty space
L lymphatics

Anterior
superior
iliac
supine

N A
V

E

Pubic
tubercule

Greater
saphenous
vein

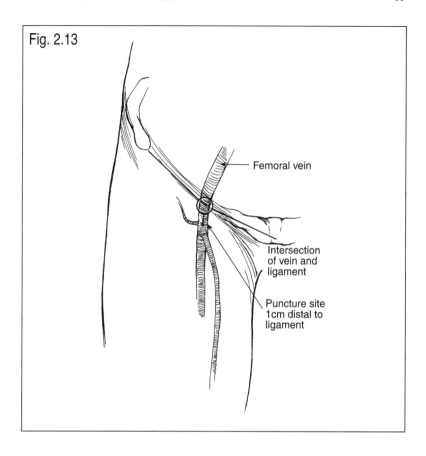

Fig. 2.13

Femoral vein

Intersection
of vein and
ligament

Puncture site
1cm distal to
ligament

i. Introduce the J wire, with the tip aimed toward the heart, through the needle while maintaining the needle in the same location. The wire must pass with minimal resistance.

j. If resistance is met, remove the wire and check needle placement by withdrawing blood with a syringe.

k. Once the wire is passed, remove the needle while keeping control of the wire at all times.

l. Enlarge the puncture site with a sterile scalpel.

m. Introduce the dilator over the wire 3–4 cm to dilate the subcutaneous tissues. Advancing the dilator the entire length can lacerate the femoral vein and is not recommended.

n. Remove the dilator and introduce the catheter over the wire to the length of 15 cm.

o. Remove the wire, aspirate blood from all ports to confirm venous placement, and flush with sterile saline. Suture the catheter to the skin and apply sterile dressing.

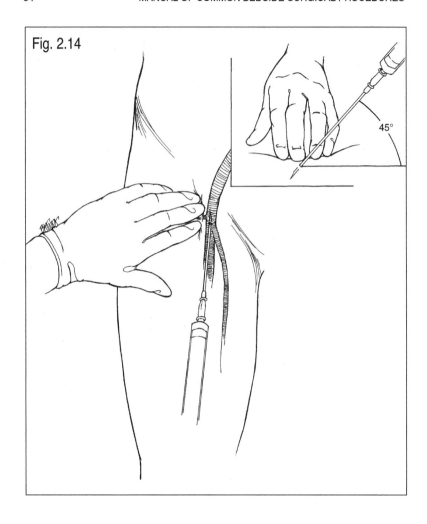

Fig. 2.14

p. Patient should maintain bed rest until the catheter is removed.

7. Complications and Management:

a. Femoral artery puncture/hematoma
- Withdraw the needle
- Hold manual pressure for at least 15–25 minutes. A
  sand bag is then placed over the site for another 30
  minutes.
- Bed rest for 4 hours
- Monitor leg pulses and site for hematoma every 30–60
  minutes.

II. OTHER VENOUS ACCESS PROCEDURES

Other forms of venous access include peripherally inserted central catheters (PICCs), which allow central venous access through a peripheral vein, tunnelled central venous catheters, and surgical access in emergent situations, such as venous cutdowns and intraosseous access. These procedures are not as commonly performed as the previously mentioned methods of venous access. Also included in this chapter is a protocol for removal of Hickman, Groshon, and other long-term indwelling venous catheters. Surgical house officers are frequently called upon to remove these devices in the outpatient clinics.

A. PERIPHERALLY INSERTED CENTRAL CATHETER, LONG ARM IV

A long, thin catheter inserted via basilic or cephalic vein to subclavian vein

1. Indications:
   a. Long-term intravenous access for drugs
   b. TPN fluids
   c. Not for CVP monitoring

2. Contraindications:
   a. Lack of upper arm veins visible or palpable with tourniquet in place
   b. Presence of phlebitis or cellulitis in arm

3. Anesthesia:
   1% lidocaine without epinephrine

4. Equipment:
   a. Most PICC kits come with everything necessary, including Betadine and alcohol swabs, sterile drapes, 3-ml syringe and 25-gauge needle, introducer (14-gauge angiographic catheter [some catheters require peel-away design]), Silastic catheter with guidewire, scissors, needle-holders, 3-0 silk suture, suture wing, gauze pads, tape measure.
   b. Equipment not contained in kits includes sterile gloves and heparinized saline for flushing catheter.

5. Positioning:

Patient should sit or recline with arm externally rotated and abducted to about 45° to axis of body. Arm should be slightly dependent with elbow extended.

6. Technique:

a. In a sterile fashion, dress with mask and gown. Place tourniquet and identify a vein in the forearm that is continuous with the basilic or cephalic vein (see Figure 2.15). Prep and drape the anticipated insertion site.

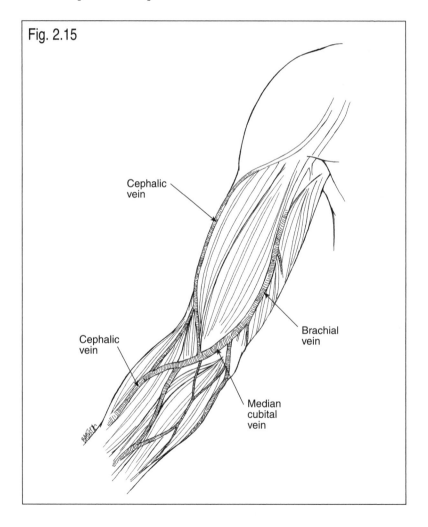

Fig. 2.15

Cephalic vein

Cephalic vein

Brachial vein

Median cubital vein

    b. Measure approximate distance to SVC from insertion site.

    c. Use a small amount of lidocaine to infiltrate skin on either side of vein.

    d. Kits that have attached hub require that the catheter be trimmed prior to insertion. Trim from the end opposite the hub (i.e., the tip). Do not trim the tip of a Groshon catheter. Flush Silastic catheter before inserting it.

    e. Place 14-gauge introducer catheter into vein as if inserting a peripheral IV. After obtaining a flash of blood, remove needle and advance plastic portion of introducer.

    f. Insert Silastic catheter through plastic introducer catheter.

    g. Remove tourniquet and advance Silastic catheter to premeasured length (some kits come with forceps to advance catheter).

    h. Remove guidewire and peel away plastic introducer catheter.

    i. Trim end of Silastic catheter to manageable length, but only if it has a detachable hub. Attach hub, heparin lock, and wings, and suture catheter to the skin. Withdraw blood and flush catheter.

    j. Confirm placement with chest radiograph.

7. Complications and Management:

    a. Bleeding
   - Apply pressure at insertion site for at least 5 minutes.

    b. Arrhythmia
   - Usually secondary to catheter being advanced too far
   - Withdraw catheter until arrhythmia resolves.
   - Medical management, if necessary

    c. Line infection
   - Suspected by positive blood cultures from the line and not from peripheral cultures.
   - Remove catheter and culture intradermal component.
   - Institute appropriate antibiotics.

    d. Clotted catheter
   - Be suspicious of intravenous clot.
   - Obtain Doppler study or venogram.
   - If clot present, line removal is recommended.

    e. Cracked or leaking catheter
   - PICCs with attachable hub can be repaired by obtaining new attachable hub, trimming catheter slightly, and placing new hub.
   - Otherwise, PICCs should be removed.

B. HOHN CATHETER

A Hohn catheter is a long-term indwelling catheter with an antibiotic-coated cuff. It is tunnelled through a short distance of the chest wall soft tissue and inserted into the subclavian vein. It is extremely flexible, with a wide lumen; successful insertion requires a two-step process, whereby a standard central line is placed and the soft-tissue tunnel is aggressively dilated prior to using Seldinger technique to rewire to the Hohn catheter.

1. Indications:
a. Long-term intravenous access for drugs
b. TPN fluids
c. Not for CVP monitoring

2. Contraindications:
a. Vein thrombosis
b. Coagulopathy (PT or PTT $> 1.5 \times$ control, platelets < 20K)
c. Untreated sepsis

3. Anesthesia:
1% lidocaine

4. Equipment:
a. Standard single-lumen central line kit, including Betadine swabs, sterile drapes, 22- and 25-gauge needles, 5-ml syringes (two), appropriate catheter and dilator, 18-gauge insertion needle (5–8 cm long), 0.035 J wire, scalpel, 2-0 silk suture.
b. Standard Hohn catheter kit, including 5-ml syringes (two), appropriate wire, and catheter.
c. Equipment not contained in kits include shoulder roll towels, mask, sterile gown, gloves, and heparinized saline for flushing catheter.

5. Positioning:
Supine, in Trendelenburg. Place a towel roll between the scapulas underneath the thoracic vertebrae. Allow the patient's shoulders to fall down and back (or have an assistant apply gentle traction to the ipsilateral arm).

6. Technique:

a. Follow the technique described previously (Section I A 6) for placing a subclavian central venous catheter using materials from a standard single-lumen central line kit.

b. After the standard central venous catheter is in position, introduce the guidewire from the Hohn catheter kit through the central venous catheter and remove the catheter over the wire (Seldinger technique).

c. While keeping control of the wire, introduce the dilator from the Hohn catheter kit over the wire 3–4 cm to further generously dilate the subcutaneous tissues.

d. Remove the dilator and introduce the Hohn catheter over the wire. A strong, persistent twisting motion around the long axis of the catheter is required to advance the large, floppy Hohn through the soft tissue. The antibiotic-coated cuff should come to rest just above the insertion site in the soft tissue tunnel.

e. Remove the wire, aspirate blood to confirm venous placement, and flush with sterile saline. Suture the Hohn catheter to the skin and apply sterile dressing.

f. Run IV fluids at 20 ml/hr and order a portable CXR to confirm placement in SVC and rule out pneumothorax.

7. Complications and Management:

a. Arterial puncture
  - Withdraw needle immediately and apply manual pressure for 5 minutes.
  - Monitor hemodynamics and breath sounds for hemothorax.

b. Air embolus
  - Attempt to withdraw air by aspirating through catheter.
  - If hemodynamically unstable (cardiac arrest), initiate ACLS protocol and thoracic surgery consultation.
  - If stable, position patient in left lateral decubitus and Trendelenburg position to trap air in right ventricle. CXR in this position can show significant air and be used for follow up.
  - Air will eventually dissolve.

c. Pneumothorax
  - If a tension pneumothorax is suspected, decompress with 16-gauge angiographic catheter in second intercostal space, midclavicular line.

- If < 10%, 100% oxygen and serial CXRs
- If > 10%, tube thoracostomy

   d. Malpositioning
  - Into RA or RV, against wall of vein—withdraw or advance as needed to place into SVC
  - Into other subclavian vein—stable position, no adjustment needed
  - Into jugular or mammary vein—re-introduce J wire, remove catheter, thread long 18-gauge angiographic catheter and confirm placement in vein by aspiration of blood. The J wire can now be redirected into SVC by maximizing positioning (pull caudally on arm and turn the head and neck in the ipsilateral direction to close internal jugular vein angle).

   e. Dysrhythmias
  - Atrial or ventricular dysrhythmias are associated with wires and catheters in the RA or RV and usually resolve after withdrawing the catheter into the SVC.
  - Persistent dysrhythmias may need medical management.

   f. Line infection (line should be removed within 6 weeks)
  - Confirmed by positive blood cultures from the line and not from peripheral cultures
  - Remove catheter and culture intradermal component.
  - Institute appropriate antibiotics.

C. HICKMAN REMOVAL

1. Indications:
   a. Infected catheter
   b. Intractably clotted catheter
   c. Completion of therapy

2. Contraindications:
   a. Severe coagulopathy (PT or PTT >1.5 × control)
   b. Continued need for therapy

3. Anesthesia:
   1% lidocaine

4. Equipment:
   a. Betadine prep solution
   b. Sterile drapes

    c. Sterile hemostats, scalpel with blade, needle holder
    d. 4-0 nylon suture

5. Positioning:

Supine

6. Technique:

a. Prep Hickman insertion site and catheter.
b. Infiltrate site with local anesthetic, including catheter tract up to and including cuff.
c. With gentle, steady pressure, pull Hickman catheter. Sometimes this is enough to dislodge cuff from surrounding fibrous tissue.
d. When cuff is close to skin incision, insert hemostat via tract to cuff site. Use blunt spreading technique to divide fibrous tissue (see Figure 2.16).
e. Occasionally it is necessary to enlarge the skin incision. Use the scalpel, taking care to avoid lacerating catheter. If necessary, make an incision directly over the cuff and then use blunt dissection to free the cuff.
f. Once the cuff is freed from the fibrous tissue, gently and steadily pull the catheter from the tract.
g. Apply pressure to the subclavian or internal jugular vein area as the tip of catheter exits the vein.
h. If skin incision is large, approximate edges with suture. Apply dressing.

7. Complications and Management:

a. Air embolus
    • Unlikely with removal of tunnelled catheter
    • If hemodynamically unstable, initiate ACLS protocol and thoracic surgery consultation.
    • If stable, place patient in left lateral decubitus and Trendelenburg position to trap air in right ventricle.
    • Follow with serial CXRs. Air will eventually dissolve.
b. Bleeding
    • Apply direct pressure for 15 minutes.
c. Catheter breakage
    • If external to skin site, prevent air embolus by clamping catheter proximal to breakage site and remove catheter.

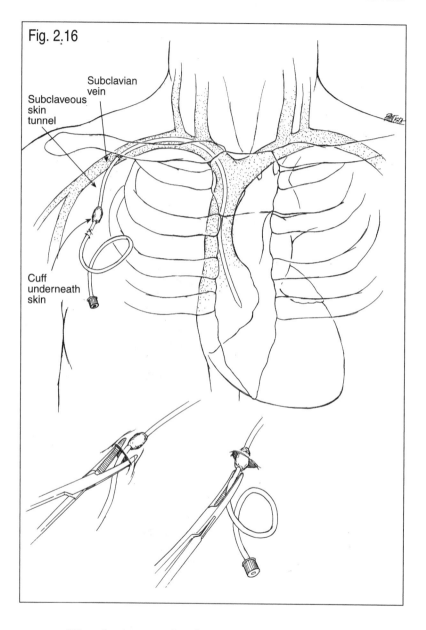

Fig. 2.16

- If break occurs under the skin and the catheter end retracts through the tunnel, interventional radiology will need to retrieve catheter.
- This is a serious complication. Avoid it by not pulling catheter too hard and by keeping sharp instruments out of the tunnel.

D. GREATER SAPHENOUS VENOUS CUTDOWN

1. Indications:

Saphenous vein cutdown is performed when percutaneous access to the venous system cannot be gained. It can be used to gain lower extremity access for trauma, but in recent years has been replaced by the percutaneous femoral vein approach. The preferred site for saphenous vein cutdown is at the ankle. Although the saphenous vein can also be reached by a cutdown in the groin, it is rarely performed as an elective bedside procedure.

2. Contraindications:
   a. Coagulopathy (PT or PTT > 1.5 × control)
   b. Vein thrombosis

3. Anesthesia:
   1% lidocaine

4. Equipment:
   a. Tourniquet
   b. Mask and sterile prep solution, gown, gloves, drape
   c. Gauze pads
   d. 3-ml syringe with 25-gauge needle
   e. Sterile scalpel, hemostat, fine scissors
   f. IV catheter and heparin lock cap
   g. 3-0 silk ties

5. Positioning:

Patient should be in position comfortable for the operator, usually supine, with extremity of interest in dependent position.

6. Technique:
   a. The greater saphenous vein is consistently located about 1 cm anterior and superior to the medial malleolus (see Figure 2.17). A tourniquet is unnecessary for access to the vein.
   b. Prep and drape area surrounding the ankle. Infiltrate the skin over the vein with lidocaine using a 25-gauge needle.
   c. Make a full-thickness transverse incision through the anesthetized skin to a length of 2.5 cm.

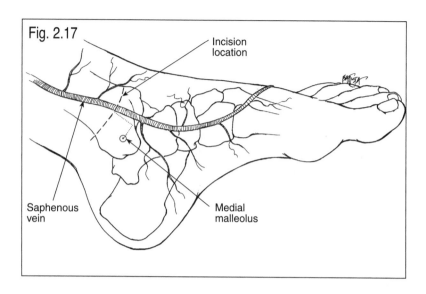

Fig. 2.17

Incision location

Saphenous vein

Medial malleolus

d. Using a curved hemostat, identify the saphenous vein and gently dissect it free from the saphenous nerve, which is attached to the anterior wall of the vein. It is imperative that the saphenous nerve be identified to avoid injury and subsequent pain.

e. Elevate and dissect the vein free from its bed for a distance of approximately 2 cm (see Figure 2.18).

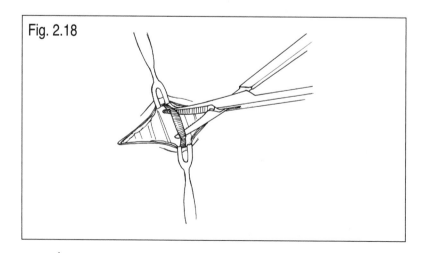

Fig. 2.18

f. Pass the silk ties around the exposed vein proximally and distally.

g. Ligate the vein distally, leaving the suture in place for traction.

h. Make a small transverse venotomy and gently dilate the venotomy with the tip of the closed hemostat. A vein introducer may also be used (see Figure 2.19).

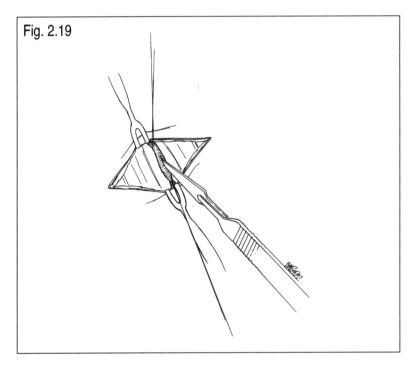

Fig. 2.19

i. Place angiographic catheter into the vein directly or after tunnelling it through the skin distal to the incision. Tie the proximal silk suture to secure the catheter, being careful not to occlude the catheter. The catheter should be inserted an adequate distance to prevent easy dislodgement (see Figure 2.20).

j. Close wound with interrupted nylon sutures. Apply sterile dressings.

7. Complications and Management:

a. Bleeding
   • Apply pressure if bleeding occurs.

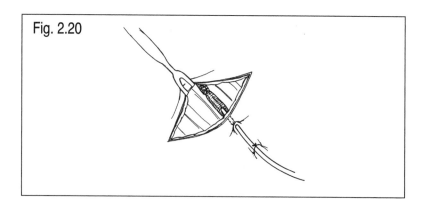

Fig. 2.20

  b. Infection/Phlebitis
    • Remove catheter. Apply warm compresses and elevate leg.
    • Use antibiotics if necessary

E. INTRAOSSEOUS ACCESS

1. Indications:

Need for emergency access, usually in a child less than 3 years old, when other attempts at venous access have failed and time is too short for a cutdown. The technique has been used in older children and adults. Once intravascular volume has been replaced, other access should be obtained.

2. Contraindications:

  a. Because this is an emergency procedure and is to be used in the severely injured or critically ill patient, the only relative contraindication is injury to the extremity of interest.
  b. Avoid placing the needle distal to a fracture site.

3. Anesthesia:

None

4. Equipment:

16- or 18-gauge bone marrow aspiration or intraosseous infusion needle

5. Positioning:

Supine

6. Technique:

a. Insert needle, bevel up, at 60°–90° angle into the marrow of a long bone. The preferred site is the tibia 2–3 cm inferior to the tibial tuberosity; alternatively, use the inferior third of the femur (see Figure 2.21).

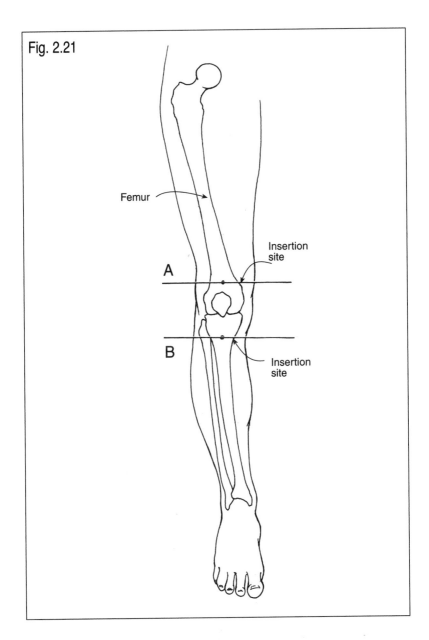

Fig. 2.21

Femur

Insertion site

A

B

Insertion site

b. Aspiration of marrow confirms proper location. Other clues to proper position include firm upright position of needle in bone and easy infusion of 5–10 ml of fluid (see Figure 2.22).
c. Secure the needle with tape.

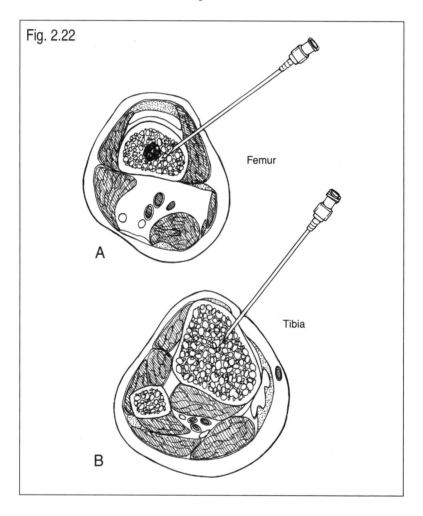

Fig. 2.22

A

Femur

Tibia

B

7. Complications and Management:
   a. Infiltration
      • Remove and replace needle.
   b. Cellulitis
      • Remove needle.
      • Treat cellulitis with antibiotics.

c. Osteomyelitis
   • Appropriate long-term IV antibiotics
d. Compartment syndrome
   • Fasciotomy

III. ARTERIAL CANNULATION

Arterial lines permit continuous monitoring of heart rate and blood pressure necessary in ICU patients who are receiving inotropic agents or who are hemodynamically unstable. Intraoperative monitoring is also required with high-risk patients. In order of preference, we attempt radial > ulnar > femoral > dorsalis pedis > axillary sites. We recommend using "quick" catheters or angiographic catheters for radial, ulnar, and dorsalis pedis arteries, and the Seldinger technique for femoral and axillary arteries.

A. RADIAL ARTERY CANNULATION

1. Indications:
   a. Continuous hemodynamic monitoring
   b. Frequent assessment of arterial blood gases

2. Contraindications:
   Allen test.
   a. Occlude both ulnar and radial arteries and allow venous drainage to exsanguinate the hand (see Figure 2.23).
   b. Release the ulnar artery while keeping the radial artery compressed.
   c. If hand color does not return in < 5 seconds, the Allen test is positive and cannulation should be aborted.

3. Anesthesia:
   1% lidocaine

4. Equipment:
   a. Sterile prep solution
   b. Mask, sterile gown, gloves, and towels
   c. 25-gauge needle

Fig. 2.23

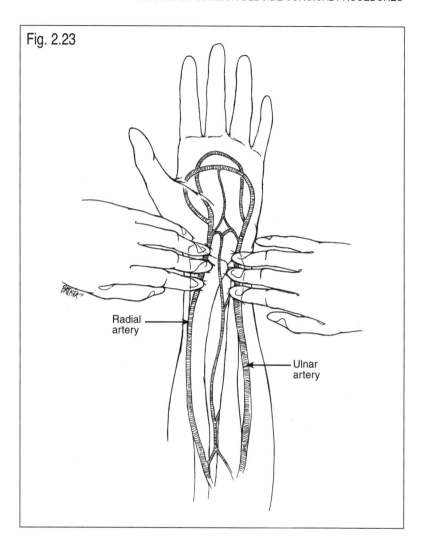

Radial artery

Ulnar artery

d. Syringe
e. 16-, 18-, or 20-gauge angiographic catheter (2 inches long)quick catheters
f. 2–0 silk sutures
g. Pressure bags with IV tubing
h. Heparinized flush system with sensor attachments for monitoring
i. Sterile dressings
j. Hand towel

5. Positioning:

Expose the ventral surface of the forearm, dorsiflex the wrist, and place a rolled-up hand towel underneath the dorsal surface of the wrist. Secure the palm and forearm to an arm board (see Figure 2.24).

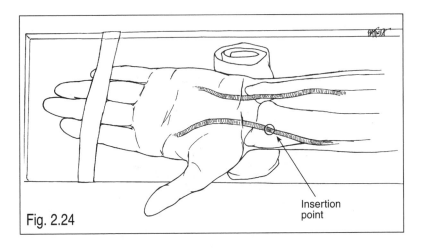

Fig. 2.24

Insertion point

6. Technique (use technique similar to ulnar artery cannulation):

a. In a sterile fashion, dress with mask and gown. Prep and drape ventral surface of the wrist.

b. Palpate the radial pulse near the distal radius.

c. Administer anesthetic with a 25-gauge needle into the skin above this point. Use a 19-gauge needle as a skin breaker to puncture the skin.

d. Using an angiographic catheter, enter at a 45° angle and advance toward the pulse until blood return is seen in the hub of the needle (see Figure 2.25).

e. If there is no blood return, withdraw the angiographic catheter slowly and make another pass at a 60° angle toward the palpated pulse.

f. If good blood return is seen in the hub, advance the angiographic catheter another 2 mm to ensure intraluminal placement of the angiographic catheter. If you are using a quick catheter, this additional 2 mm is not necessary and the wire portion of the system is then advanced into the artery.

g. Slowly advance the catheter portion of the angiographic catheter into the artery while holding the needle steady.

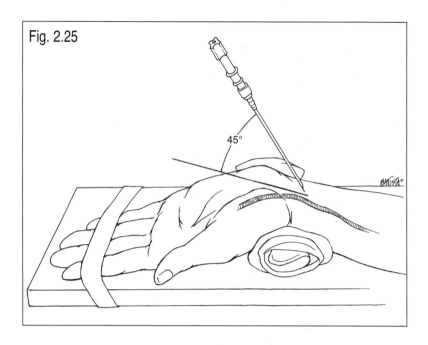

Fig. 2.25

45°

h. Remove the needle and keep digital compression on the proximal radial artery to prevent excessive bleeding.
i. If there is no bleeding, the catheter is not intraluminal. Withdraw the catheter slowly in case it has punctured the posterior wall. If there is still no blood, remove the catheter, hold pressure for 5 minutes. Reassess landmarks and reattempt placement. Often the artery lies more medially than expected.
j. If successful, attach flush system and sensors to the monitor to assess arterial waveform.
k. Suture the catheter to the skin and apply sterile dressing.
l. If unsuccessful after three attempts, stop and assess a more proximal site.

7. Complications and Management:
   a. Poor arterial waveform
      • Check all line connections and stopcocks.
      • Exclude extrinsic proximal arterial compression.
      • Check position of arm and wrist; the arm cannot be elevated and the wrist must be dorsiflexed.
      • If waveform and blood return are poor, replace catheter.
   b. Ischemic digits
      • Remove catheter and monitor the hand.

B. DORSALIS PEDIS ARTERY CANNULATION

1. Indications:
   a. Continuous hemodynamic monitoring
   b. Frequent assessment of arterial blood gases

2. Contraindications:

   No palpable dorsalis pedis artery

3. Anesthesia:

   1% lidocaine

4. Equipment:
   a. Sterile prep solution
   b. Mask, sterile gown, gloves, and towels
   c. 25-gauge needle
   d. 5-ml syringe
   e. 16-, 18-, or 20-gauge angiographic catheter (2 inches long) or quick catheters
   f. 2–0 silk sutures
   g. Pressure bags with IV tubing
   h. Heparinized flush system with sensor attachments for monitoring
   i. Sterile dressings

5. Positioning:

   Expose the dorsal surface of the foot in neutral position.

6. Technique:
   a. In a sterile fashion, dress with mask and gown. Prep and drape dorsal surface of the foot.
   b. Palpate the dorsalis pedis pulse lateral to the extensor hallucis longus at the level of the metatarsal–1st cuneiform joint (see Figure 2.26), and administer anesthetic with a 25-gauge needle into the skin above this point.
   c. Using a 20-gauge angiographic catheter with the bevel up, puncture the skin at a 45° angle to the skin. Advance the angiographic catheter toward the palpated pulse until blood return is seen in the hub of the needle (see Figure 2.27).

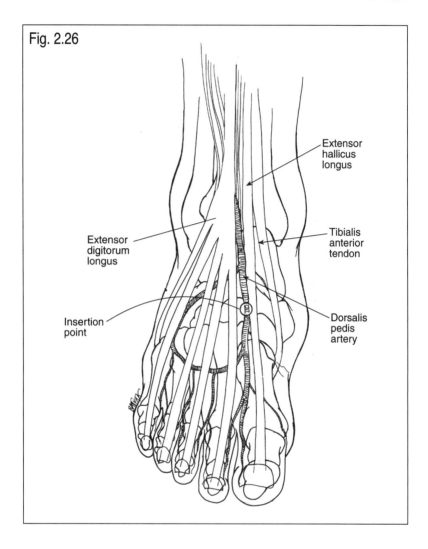

Fig. 2.26

Extensor
hallicus
longus

Tibialis
anterior
tendon

Extensor
digitorum
longus

Dorsalis
pedis
artery

Insertion
point

d. If there is no blood return, withdraw angiographic catheter
slowly and make another pass at a 60° angle toward the palpated pulse.

e. If there is good blood return in the hub, advance the angiographic catheter another 2 mm to ensure intraluminal placement. If you are using a quick catheter, this additional 2 mm
is unnecessary and the wire portion of the system is advanced into the artery.

f. While maintaining a firm hold on the needle portion of the
angiographic catheter, slowly advance the catheter portion
into the artery.

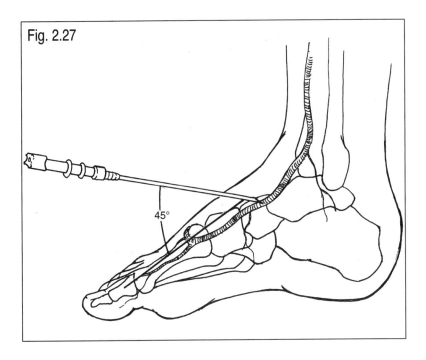

Fig. 2.27

45°

g. Remove the needle and keep digital compression proximally to prevent excessive bleeding.
h. If there is no bleeding, the catheter is not intraluminal. Withdraw the catheter slowly in case it has punctured the posterior wall. If there is still no blood, remove the catheter and hold pressure for 5 minutes. Reassess landmarks and reattempt placement.
i. If successful, attach flush system and sensors to the monitor to assess arterial waveform.
j. Suture the catheter to the skin and apply a sterile dressing.
k. If unsuccessful after three attempts, stop and assess another site.

7. Complications and Management:
   a. Poor arterial waveform
      • Check all line connections and stopcocks.
      • Exclude extrinsic proximal arterial compression.
      • If waveform and blood return are poor, replace catheter.
   b. Ischemic toes
      • Remove catheter and monitor foot.

C. FEMORAL ARTERY CANNULATION

1. Indications:
   a. Continuous hemodynamic monitoring
   b. Frequent assessment of arterial blood gases
   c. Access for arteriography studies
   d. Intra-aortic balloon pump insertion (see Chapter 3)

2. Contraindications:
   a. Prior groin surgery (relative)
   b. Patient should maintain bed rest while catheter is in place.

3. Anesthesia:

   1% lidocaine

4. Equipment:
   a. Sterile prep solution
   b. Mask, sterile gown, gloves, and towels
   c. 25-gauge needle
   d. 5-ml syringes (two)
   e. 16-gauge catheter (6 inches)
   f. 18-gauge insertion needle (5 cm long)
   g. 0.035 J wire, sterile dressings
   h. Safety razor
   i. 2–0 silk sutures
   j. Pressure bags with IV tubing
   k. Heparinized flush system with sensor attachments for monitoring

5. Positioning:

   Supine

6. Technique:
   a. In a sterile fashion, dress with mask and gown. Shave, prep, and drape left or right groin area.
   b. Palpate the femoral pulse at the midpoint along an imaginary line between the anterior superior iliac spine and the symphysis pubis. Palpate its course 1–2 cm distally.

c. Administer anesthetic with 25-gauge needle into the skin and subcutaneous tissues along the course of the artery (see Figure 2.28).

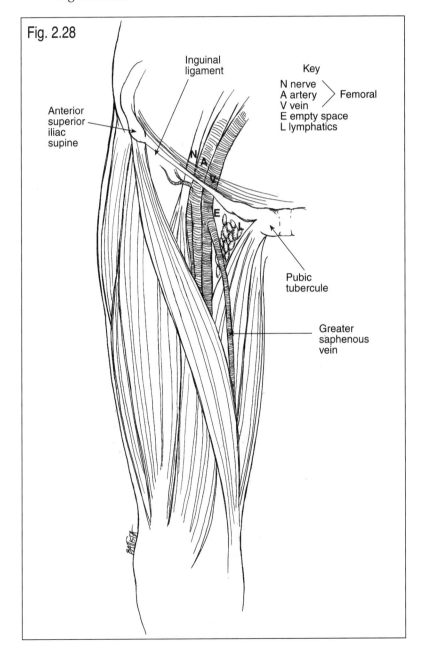

Fig. 2.28

Inguinal ligament

Key

N nerve
A artery } Femoral
V vein
E empty space
L lymphatics

Anterior superior iliac supine

Pubic tubercule

Greater saphenous vein

d. Using the 18-gauge insertion needle with a 5-ml syringe, puncture the skin at point A and advance the needle while aspirating cranially at a 45° angle to the skin toward the pulse (see Figures 2.29 and 2.30).

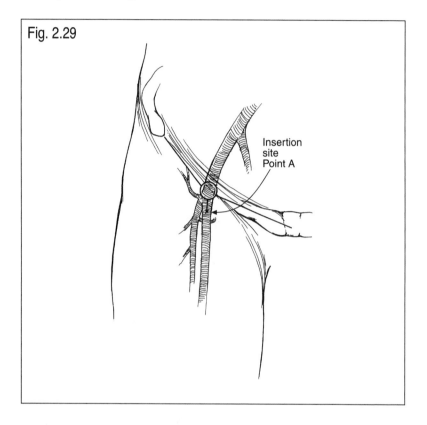

Fig. 2.29

Insertion site
Point A

e. If there is no arterial blood return after 5 cm, slowly withdraw needle while aspirating. If still no return, redirect again toward the pulse or reassess landmarks and attempt access at a site that is 1 cm more proximal along the course of the artery.
f. If there is venous return, withdraw needle and hold pressure according to the complications section.
g. If arterial access is obtained, remove the syringe while keeping a finger over the needle to prevent excessive bleeding.
h. Introduce the J wire, with the tip aimed toward the heart, through the needle (Seldinger technique). The wire must pass with minimal resistance.

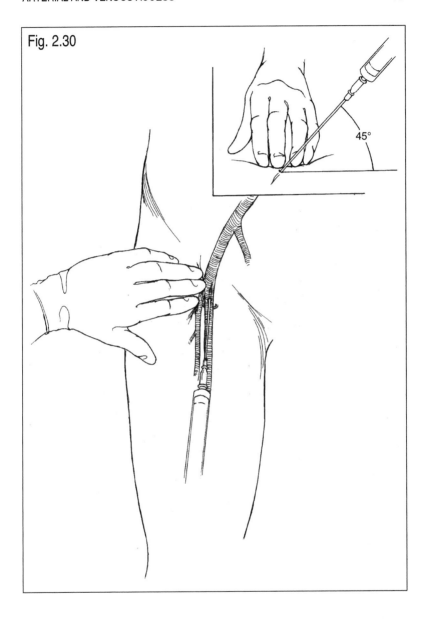

Fig. 2.30

45°

i. If resistance is met, remove the wire and check needle placement by withdrawing blood with a syringe.
j. Once the wire is passed, remove the needle while keeping control of the wire at all times.
k. Enlarge the puncture site carefully with a sterile scalpel.
l. Introduce the catheter over the wire.

m. Remove the wire and attach flush system and sensors to the monitor to assess arterial waveform. Suture the catheter to the skin and apply a sterile dressing.

n. Patient should maintain bed rest until the catheter is removed.

7. Complications and Management:
   a. Femoral vein puncture
      • Withdraw the needle.
      • Hold pressure for 10 minutes.
   b. Thrombosis
      • Remove catheter.
      • Closely monitor leg pulses and observe for distal emboli.
   c. Hematoma
      • Remove catheter.
      • Hold pressure for at least 15 minutes. A sand bag is then placed over the site for another 30 minutes.
      • Bed rest for 4 hours.
      • Monitor leg pulses.

D. AXILLARY ARTERY CANNULATION

1. Indications:
   a. Continuous hemodynamic monitoring
   b. Frequent assessment of arterial blood gases
   c. Access for arteriography studies

2. Contraindications:
   a. Unable to abduct arm
   b. Poor distal peripheral pulses

3. Anesthesia:
   1% lidocaine

4. Equipment:
   a. Sterile prep solution
   b. Mask and sterile gown, gloves, and towels
   c. 25-gauge needle
   d. 5-ml syringes (two)
   e. 16-gauge catheter (6 inches)
   f. 18-gauge insertion needle (5 cm long)
   g. 0.035 J wire
   h. Sterile dressings

  i. Safety razor
  j. 2–0 silk sutures
  k. Pressure bags with IV tubing
  l. Heparinized flush system with sensor attachments for monitoring

5. Positioning:

 Supine with the shoulder externally rotated and the arm fully abducted

6. Technique:

  a. In a sterile fashion, dress with mask and gown. Shave, prep, and drape axilla.
  b. Palpate the axillary pulse as proximally as possible inferior to the pectoralis major.
  c. Administer anesthetic with 25-gauge needle into the skin and subcutaneous tissues along the course of the artery (see Figure 2.31).

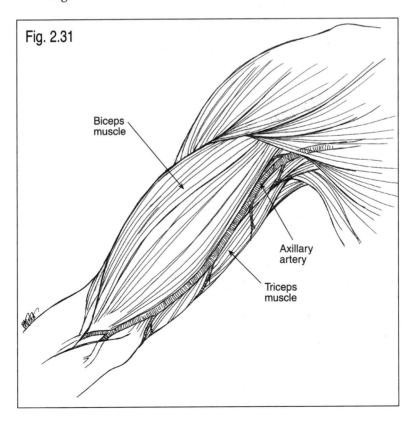

Fig. 2.31

Biceps muscle

Axillary artery

Triceps muscle

d. Using the 18-gauge insertion needle with a 5-ml syringe, puncture the skin and advance the needle while aspirating at a 45° angle to the skin toward the pulse (see Figure 2.32).

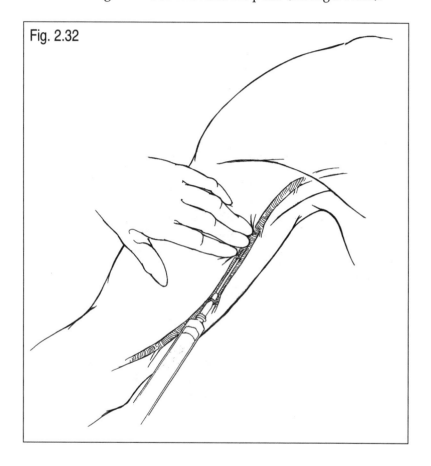

Fig. 2.32

e. If there is no arterial return after 5 cm, slowly withdraw needle while aspirating and redirect toward the pulse. If there is still no return, reassess landmarks and attempt access at a site that is 1 cm more distal along the course of the artery.
f. If venous blood is encountered, withdraw needle and hold pressure according to the complications section.
g. If arterial access is obtained, remove the syringe while keeping a finger over the needle to prevent excessive bleeding.
h. Introduce the J wire through the needle with the tip aimed toward the heart, while maintaining the needle in the same location. The wire must pass with minimal resistance.

    i. If resistance is met, remove the wire and check needle placement by withdrawing blood with a syringe.

    j. Once the wire is passed, remove the needle while keeping control of the wire at all times.

    k. Enlarge the puncture site carefully with a sterile scalpel.

    l. Introduce the catheter over the wire.

    m. Remove the wire and attach flush system and sensors to the monitor to assess arterial waveform. Suture the catheter to the skin and apply sterile dressing.

7. Complications and Management:

    a. Venous puncture
- Withdraw needle.
- Hold pressure for at least 10 minutes.

    b. Thrombosis
- Remove catheter.
- Monitor distal pulses and watch for ischemic digits.

    c. Brachial plexus injury
- Remove catheter.
- Assess neurological function. If no improvement, initiate neurosurgery consultation.

CHAPTER

CARDIAC PROCEDURES

Authors: Sunjay Kaushal, M.D., Ph.D., and Jorge D. Salazar, M.D.

CARDIAC PROCEDURES

I. CARDIAC PROCEDURES

Cardiac procedures play an important role in the care of medical and surgical patients. These procedures are life-saving maneuvers that should be familiar to every house officer. Additionally, the surgical house staff should be able to perform more invasive techniques such as pericardiocentesis, pulmonary artery catheter placement, and intra-aortic balloon pump (IABP) placement.

A. DEFIBRILLATION/CARDIOVERSION

1. Indications:
    a. For defibrillation
        • Ventricular fibrillation (VF)
        • Pulseless ventricular tachycardia (VT)
    b. Cardioversion
        • Any hemodynamically unstable tachyarrhythmia other than VF or pulseless VT (e.g., atrial fibrillation, atrial flutter, or other super ventricular tachycardias)
        • Elective conversion in patients with stable tachyarrhythmias

2. Contraindications:
    None

3. Anesthesia:
    If time and the patient's blood pressure permit, one may give a sedative (e.g., diazepam, midazolam, ketamine) with

or without an analgesic agent (e.g., fentanyl, morphine). See Appendix C.

4. Equipment:
   a. Electrode gel
   b. Defibrillator
   c. Electrocardiograph (ECG) machine with three-lead rhythm
   d. Central line IV access

5. Positioning:
   a. Place the patient in a supine position away from water or metal surfaces.
   b. Expose the entire chest and remove any transdermal patches.

6. Technique:
   The procedure for electroconvulsion should follow the ACLS protocols described in Appendix A, and the technique is described below.
   a. Apply gel to hand-held paddles, or use adhesive electrode pads.
   b. Turn on machine. Set to defibrillate (asynchronous) for VF or pulseless VT or cardiovert (synchronous) for all other arrhythmias. See chart below.

	Defibrillate	Cardiovert
Mode	Asynchronous	Synchronous
Arrhythmia	VT or VF	Other unstable arrhythmias
First shock	200 J	50 or 100 J
Second shock	300 J	200 J
Third shock	360 J	300 or 360 J

   c. Set machine to the appropriate energy level. The first shock should be 200 J for defibrillation and 50 or 100 J for electroconvulsion.
   d. Charge the capacitor.
   e. Place electrodes on chest. There are two acceptable placements:
      • One electrode to the right of the upper sternum and the other over the apex of the heart to the left of the nipple in the midaxillary line (see Figure 3.1)

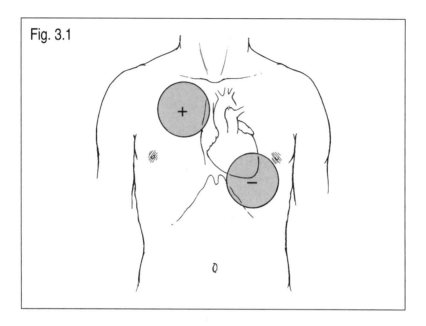

Fig. 3.1

- One electrode anteriorly over the left precordium (A) and the other posteriorly beneath the left scapula (B) (see Figure 3.2)
- Avoid positioning electrodes over pacemakers.

f. Apply firm pressure, about 25 pounds, to the hand-held paddles. Announce that defibrillation/cardioversion is about to occur and loudly state "All clear!"

g. Ensure that no person is in contact with the patient or bed.

h. Deliver an electric shock by pressing both discharge buttons simultaneously.

i. If the initial rhythm persists, repeat shock at the next level up to a maximum of 360 J. If still no success, CPR should continue with intubation and intravenous access. The use of pharmacotherapy should be initiated per ACLS protocol.

7. Complications and Management:

a. Inadvertent shock to bystanders
- Usually results in temporary discomfort to the recipient, but may involve serious burns.
- The best treatment is prevention.

b. Temporary or permanent pacemaker malfunction
- After the patient is successfully resuscitated and hemodynamically stable, it may be necessary to interrogate

Fig. 3.2

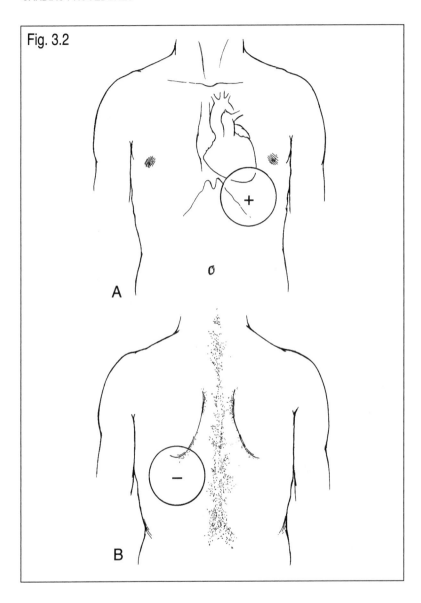

and/or reset the pacemaker and consult cardiology service.
- Place a transcutaneous pacer or insert a temporary transvenous pacer, if needed (see Section C).
c. Cutaneous burns
- Usually only first-degree burns, but may extend deeper.
- Treat according to depth of burn.

B. PERICARDIOCENTESIS

1. Indications:
   a. To prevent further cardiac compression due to cardiac tamponade, which is manifested by increased intracardiac pressures, reduction of ventricular diastolic filling, and/or decrease in cardiac output or stroke volume
   b. To establish a diagnosis from pericardial fluid

2. Contraindications:
   a. Coagulopathy (platelets < 50,000, PT or PTT > 1.3 × control)
   b. Post—coronary bypass surgery because of risk of injury to grafts
   c. Acute traumatic hemopericardium
   d. Small pericardial effusion, less than 200 ml
   e. Absence of an anterior effusion or if effusion is loculated

3. Anesthesia:
   1% lidocaine

4. Equipment:
   a. Sterile prep solution
   b. Sterile gloves and towels
   c. Long 3-inch 16- or 18-gauge needle
   d. 16-gauge Teflon catheter
   e. 30-ml syringe
   f. ECG monitor
   g. Sterile alligator connector
   h. 0.035-cm J wire
   i. 2-0 nylon suture
   j. Safety razor
   k. Scalpel and #11 blade

5. Positioning:
   Supine with the head of the bed elevated 30° to allow dependent pooling of blood or effusion to the area to be aspirated.

6. Technique:
   a. Sterile prep and drape the chest and subxiphoid area.
   b. Identify the needle entry site 0.5 cm immediately left of the xiphoid tip (see Figure 3.3).

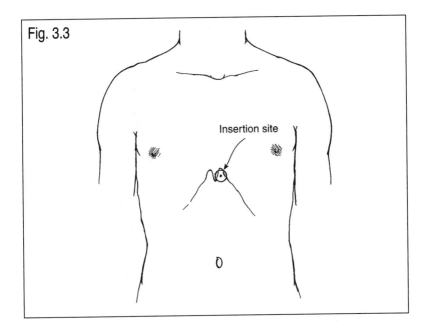

Fig. 3.3

Insertion site

c. Administer 1% lidocaine with a 25-gauge needle into the skin and subcutaneous tissue in this area, always aspirating before injecting.

d. Insert the long 3-inch 16- or 18-gauge needle attached to a syringe through the anesthetized skin 0.5 cm immediately left of the xiphoid tip.

e. Attach a precordial limb lead of the ECG machine to the needle with an alligator clip for monitoring.

f. Advance the needle through the skin at a 45° angle to the thorax (underneath the sternum) and directed posteriorly, aiming toward the left shoulder. Apply continuous aspiration (see Figure 3.4).

g. Negative deflection of the QRS complex will be seen when contact is made with the epicardium of the pericardial sac (see Figure 3.5).

h. Advance the needle (a few centimeters) further through the epicardium into the pericardial space. Nonclotting blood or effusion may be encountered. ST segment elevation indicates contact with the myocardium. Withdraw the needle into the pericardial space, where no ST segment elevation should be seen.

i. Aspirate all fluid present.

j. For continuous drainage, a 16-gauge soft Teflon catheter may be placed via the Seldinger technique as follows.

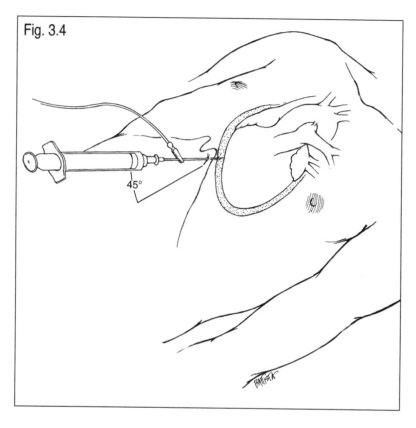

Fig. 3.4

45°

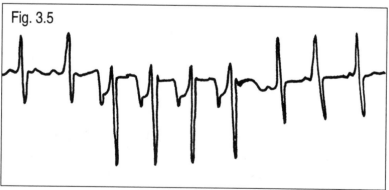

Fig. 3.5

k. Insert the J wire through the needle into the pericardial space.
l. Remove the needle, leaving the wire in place.
m. Enlarge the skin incision to about 0.3 cm with a scalpel.
n. Pass the catheter over the wire into the pericardial space (see Figure 3.6).

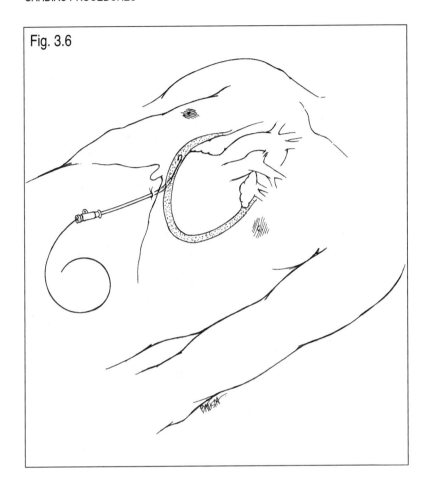

Fig. 3.6

o. Remove the wire and attach the catheter to a closed-system drainage bag.
p. Suture the catheter to the skin.
q. If pericardiocentesis is performed for diagnostic purposes, send fluid for cell count analysis; measurement of amylase, protein, and glucose; and culture of anaerobic or aerobic bacteria, acid-fast bacilli, or fungi.
r. Monitor the patient for 24 hours in an intensive care setting for recurrence of pericardial effusion.
s. Obtain an ECG for documentation of the function and appearance of the heart and pericardium.
t. Success in reducing tamponade is measured by a decrease in right atrial pressures, an increase in cardiac output, and a disappearance of pulsus paradoxus.

7. Complications and Management:

a. Cardiac puncture or laceration of a coronary artery
- Monitor vital signs and ECG closely.
- May require emergent thoracotomy or sternotomy

b. Air embolus
- Attempt to withdraw air by aspirating through catheter.
- If hemodynamically unstable (cardiac arrest), initiate ACLS and obtain a thoracic surgery consultation.
- If stable, position patient in left lateral decubitus and Trendelenburg position to trap air in right ventricle. CXR in this position can demonstrate significant air entrapment and serial x-rays should be obtained to follow the air embolus. Eventually, the air embolus should dissolve.

c. Cardiac arrhythmias
- Withdraw needle if hemodynamically significant.
- May require pharmacotherapy or electroconvulsion per ACLS protocol

d. Hemothorax or pneumothorax
- Monitor with serial CXRs.
- If significant, tube thoracostomy (see Chapter 4)

e. Infection
- Catheter should be left in place for a maximum of 48 hours.
- Antibiotics if appropriate

C. TEMPORARY TRANSVENOUS CARDIAC PACING

1. Indications:

a. Perioperative management of cardiac surgery patients
b. Short-term treatment of arrhythmias and heart block
c. High risk of developing third-degree AV block
d. Sick sinus syndrome
e. Asystole in acute myocardial infarction

2. Contraindications:

a. Severe hypothermia
- Bradycardia may be physiological in hypothermic patients. As the patient's temperature decreases, the heart becomes more irritable, creating potential for fibrillation when paced.
b. Cardiac arrest for more than 20 minutes (low likelihood of successful resuscitation with such a prolonged arrest)

3. Anesthesia:

 A sedative agent and an analgesic (see Appendix C)

4. Equipment:
    a. Sterile prep solution
    b. Sterile gloves and towels
    c. 22- and 25-gauge needles
    d. 5-ml syringes (two)
    e. Shoulder roll towels
    f. Appropriate catheters (percutaneous sheath introducer kit) and dilator
    g. IV tubing and flush
    h. 18-gauge insertion needle (5–8 cm long)
    i. 0.035 J wire
    j. Sterile dressings
    k. Scalpel
    l. 2-0 silk suture
    m. Pacer catheter
    n. ECG monitor
    o. Alligator clips

5. Positioning:

 Supine in Trendelenburg position and shoulder roll for subclavian vein approach.

6. Technique:
    a. Insert a 8.5-Fr cordis central venous catheter sheath into internal jugular (IJ) vein or subclavian vein per Chapter 2, Section I.
    b. Attach ECG lead V with the alligator clip to the distal lead of the pacing catheter.
    c. Gently advance the pacing catheter through the cordis into the IJ or subclavian vein using sterile technique (see Figure 3.7).
    d. As the tip of the catheter enters the right atrium, the P wave on the ECG monitor will become very large.
    e. As the tip of the catheter enters the right ventricle, the QRS complex on the ECG monitor will enlarge.
    f. ST segment elevation indicates desired placement of the pacing catheter tip against the right ventricular wall.
    g. Secure the catheter in this position by suturing it to the cordis and to the skin.

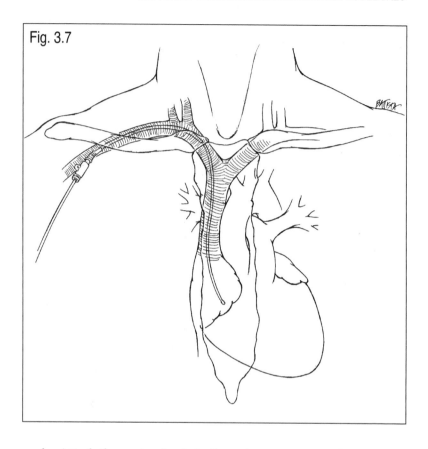

Fig. 3.7

h. Attach the pacing leads to the pulse generator and set pacer to VDD mode.
i. Obtain a CXR to confirm position.

7. Complications and Management:
   a. Lead-electrode catheter displacement
      • Usually manifested by loss of capture or sensing
      • Obtain CXR.
      • When displacement is recognized, the catheter should be immediately repositioned or removed and a new pacing catheter inserted if needed.
   b. Infection
      • Remove catheter and culture.
      • Start systemic antibiotics.
      • If pacing is necessary, insert a new catheter at a new site.
   c. Thrombosis
      • Remove the catheter and reinsert at a new site.

    d. Diaphragmatic stimulation
- May compromise ventilation.
- Reposition the catheter tip to minimize stimulation.

    e. Pneumothorax
- If a tension pneumothorax is suspected, decompress with 16-gauge IV into second intercostal space, midclavicular line and followed by tube thoracostomy.
- If < 10%, 100% oxygen and serial 4-hour CXR
- If > 10%, tube thoracostomy

D. PULMONARY ARTERY OR SWAN–GANZ CATHETER

1. Indications:

a. Evaluation of volume status in critically ill patients to determine further therapeutic interventions (fluid, vasoactive agents, assisted circulation and ventilation, emergency cardiac pacing)
b. Monitoring hemodynamic parameters in patients with low cardiac output syndromes or severe congestive heart failure (especially after open heart surgery)

2. Contraindications:

a. Vein thrombosis
b. Coagulopathy (PT or PTT > 1.3 ratio, platelets < 20,000)
c. Untreated, ongoing sepsis
d. Severe pulmonary hypertension

3. Anesthesia:

1% lidocaine

4. Equipment:

a. Sterile prep solution
b. Sterile gloves and towels
c. 22- and 25-gauge needles
d. 5-ml syringes (two)
e. Shoulder roll towels
f. Cordis catheter and dilator (sheath introducer kit)
g. IV tubing and flush
h. 18-gauge insertion needle (5–8 cm long)
i. 0.035 J wire
j. Sterile dressings

 k. Scalpel handle and #11 blade
 l. 2–0 silk suture
 m. Swan-Ganz catheter kit

5. Positioning:

Supine in Trendelenburg position, shoulder roll for subclavian vein approach

6. Technique:

 a. A cordis sheath introducer should be inserted first into one of the IJ or subclavian veins using the sterile Seldinger technique. The ideal sites for placement of the catheter are in the following order: right IJ vein, left subclavian vein, left IJ vein, and right subclavian vein. Only in critical situations should a pulmonary artery (PA) catheter be placed in the groin due to risk of infection. See Chapter 2, Section I.

 b. When the insertion site is prepped and draped, the catheter should be removed from its container and tested.

 c. Test the balloon by inflating and deflating it with the appropriate volume of air (usually 1.5 ml). Look for air leaks (see Figure 3.8).

 d. In succession, flush each of the two ports (proximal, distal) with sterile saline. Some catheters may have an additional port that requires flushing. Connect the pressure monitoring line to the transducer and confirm the waveform on the monitor by gently moving the catheter tip and watching for appropriate deflections on the monitor.

 e. Place a sterile plastic sheath over the catheter.

 f. Pass a catheter (with the balloon deflated) into the subclavian or IJ vein via the cordis by using the natural curve of the catheter to dictate the position.

 g. When the catheter has been inserted a distance of 20 cm (according to the ruler on the catheter itself), inflate the balloon with 1.5 ml of air. Do not overinflate the balloon.

 h. Gently advance the catheter with the balloon inflated into the SVC or right atrium. A CVP waveform should appear on the monitor.

 i. Continue advancing the catheter. Progression of the tip through the RV (about 40 cm) and PA (about 50 cm) will be manifested by the appropriate waveforms (Figures 3.9 and 3.10).

 j. When the catheter reaches a wedged position, the waveform will dampen.

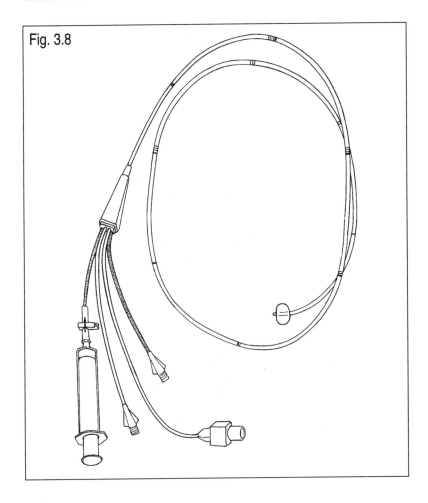

Fig. 3.8

k. When this occurs, the balloon should be deflated and a PA tracing should appear. Leave the balloon deflated when the desired position is achieved.
l. If the RV or PA tracing has not appeared after 60–70 cm, deflate the balloon, withdraw the catheter to 20 cm, inflate the balloon, and attempt another insertion. Any time the catheter needs to be withdrawn, the balloon should be deflated. Any time the catheter needs to be advanced, the balloon should be inflated.

7. Complications and Management:
   a. Pulmonary infarction from "overwedging" the catheter
      • Such a complication can be avoided by pulling the catheter

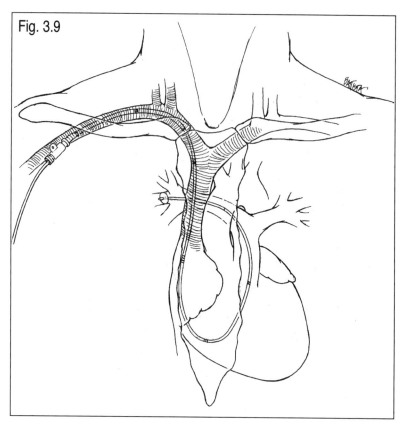

Fig. 3.9

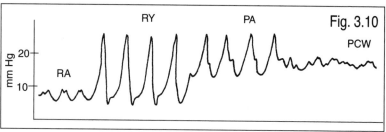

Fig. 3.10

back when the pulmonary artery phasic pressures become dampened on the monitor.

- Daily CXRs are recommended to monitor the catheter tip position.
- The balloon should not be inflated for more than 1–2 minutes at a time.
- Supply oxygenation and ventilatory support if needed.

b. Arrhythmias
  - Arrhythmias usually occur as the tip passes through the right ventricle.
  - Typically these consist of only several premature ventricular contractions (PVCs) or short runs of VT, which cease once the tip enters the PA. If, however, they persist and are hemodynamically compromising, the catheter may need to be removed and ACLS initiated.
  - Check proper position to ensure the catheter is not curled in the right ventricle.
  - Supply medical therapy if arrhythmias do not stop after catheter removal.
c. Balloon rupture
  - Leakage of 0.8–1.5 ml of air into the circulation can occur if the balloon breaks. In the pulmonary circulation this can cause pulmonary infarction. If the foramen ovale is patent and the balloon ruptures on insertion into the right heart, the air embolus could enter a coronary or cerebral artery with resultant myocardial infarction or stroke.
  - If hemodynamically unstable (cardiac arrest), initiate ACLS and obtain thoracic surgery consultation.
  - If stable, position patient in left lateral decubitus and Trendelenburg position to trap air in right ventricle. CXR in this position can show significant air and be used for follow up.
  - Air will eventually dissolve.
d. Pneumothorax
  - If a tension pneumothorax is suspected, decompress with 16-gauge IV into second intercostal space, midclavicular line followed by tube thoracostomy.
  - If < 10%, 100% oxygen and serial 4-hour CXR
  - If > 10%, tube thoracostomy
e. Rupture of the pulmonary artery
  - Pulmonary artery rupture is frequently fatal. It can be prevented by avoiding "overwedging".
  - Emergent cardiac surgery
f. Knotting of the catheter
  - The catheter may become coiled during advancement or withdrawal. If any resistance is met during positioning of the catheter, the attempt should be aborted and a CXR obtained to verify position.
  - Fluoroscopy may be needed to uncoil the catheter.

g. Infection
- The incidence of infection is increased by frequent catheter manipulation and leaving the catheter in place for more than 3 days.
- Treatment requires removal of the catheter, culture, and administration of intravenous antibiotics at times.

E. INTRA-AORTIC BALLOON PUMP

1. Indications:
   a. Cardiogenic shock
   b. Refractory left ventricular failure
   c. Mechanical complications of acute myocardial infarction (MI) (ventricular septal defect [VSD], papillary muscle dysfunction or rupture)
   d. Unstable angina refractory to medical management
   e. Ischemia-induced ventricular arrhythmias
   f. Support during percutaneous transluminal coronary angioplasty (PTCA)
   g. Weaning from cardiopulmonary bypass
   h. Bridge to transplantation

2. Contraindications:
   a. Irreversible brain damage
   b. Chronic end-stage heart disease
   c. Dissecting thoracic or aortic aneurysm
   d. Aortic insufficiency
   e. Severe peripheral vascular disease (calcified aortoiliac or femoral artery)

3. Anesthesia:
   1% lidocaine

4. Equipment:
   a. Sterile prep solution
   b. Sterile gloves and towels
   c. Angiographic needle*
   d. Guidewire*
   e. Scalpel handle and #11 blade
   f. Arterial dilator*

g. Tissue clamp
h. Sterile saline
i. Lubricant
j. IABP catheter*
k. Arterial pressure monitoring system
l. IABP system*
m. 2-0 silk suture
n. Transparent sterile tape or dressing
o. Safety razor
p. 0.035 J wire
q. Whenever possible, fluoroscopy should be used during insertion to ensure proper balloon placement.
(*contained in most IABP insertion kits)

5. Positioning:

Supine and in a monitored setting

6. Technique—Insertion:

a. Shave, sterile prep, and drape the left or right groin area.
b. Palpate the femoral pulse at the midpoint along an imaginary line between the anterior superior iliac spine and the symphysis pubis. Palpate its course 1–2 cm distally (see Figure 3.11).
c. Administer anesthetic with 25-gauge needle into the skin and subcutaneous area along the course of the artery palpated above.
d. Using the 18-gauge insertion needle with a 5-ml syringe, puncture the skin at point A and advance the needle cranially while aspirating at a 45° angle to the skin toward the pulse (see Figure 3.12).
e. If no arterial blood return after 5 cm, slowly withdraw needle while aspirating. If still no return, redirect again toward palpated pulse.
f. If still no blood return, reassess landmarks and attempt access 1 cm more proximal along the course of the artery as in Section d. If still unsuccessful, stop.
g. If venous blood encountered, withdraw needle, hold manual pressure according to the complications section, and reinsert 1 cm laterally.
h. If arterial access obtained, remove the syringe while keeping a finger over the needle to prevent excessive bleeding.
i. Introduce the J wire, with the tip aimed toward the heart, through the needle while maintaining the needle in the same

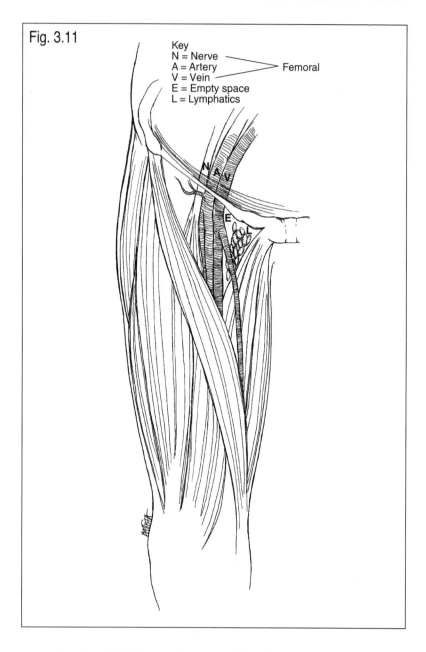

Fig. 3.11

Key
N = Nerve
A = Artery　　　　Femoral
V = Vein
E = Empty space
L = Lymphatics

location (Seldinger technique). The wire must pass with minimal resistance.
j. If resistance is met, remove the wire and check needle placement by withdrawing blood with a syringe.

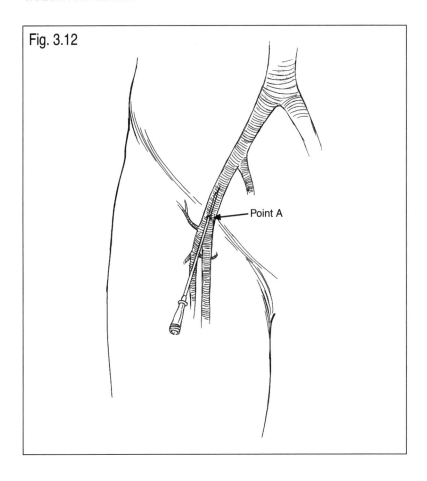

Fig. 3.12

Point A

k. Once the wire is passed, remove the needle while keeping control of the wire at all times.
l. Enlarge the puncture site carefully with a sterile scalpel.
m. Place the dilator over the J wire. Advance it through the skin into the arterial lumen. Remove the dilator.
n. Using the tissue clamp, spread the subcutaneous tissue at the insertion site.
o. Remove the IABP catheter from the kit and lubricate it with sterile saline.
p. Remove the inner stylet (see Figure 3.13).
q. Advance the IABP over the guidewire. The proper position of the catheter is with the balloon tip approximately 2 cm distal to the take off of the left subclavian artery in the descending thoracic aorta (see Figure 3.14).

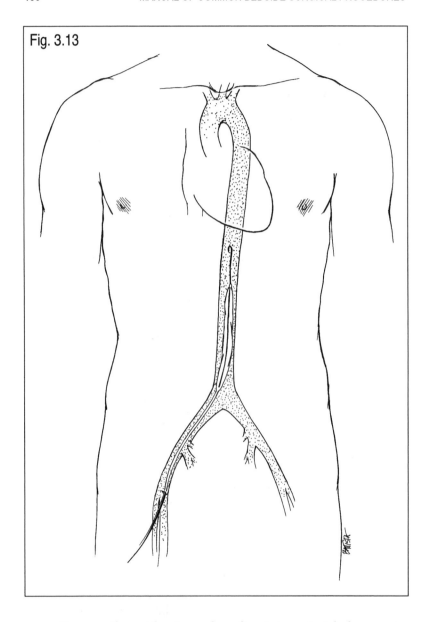

Fig. 3.13

r. Remove the guidewire and confirm intra-arterial placement by aspirating blood.
s. Attach catheter (female Luer) to a standard arterial pressure monitoring system.
t. Attach catheter (male Luer) to IABP system.
u. Suture the catheter in place. Secure and cover with clear sterile tape.

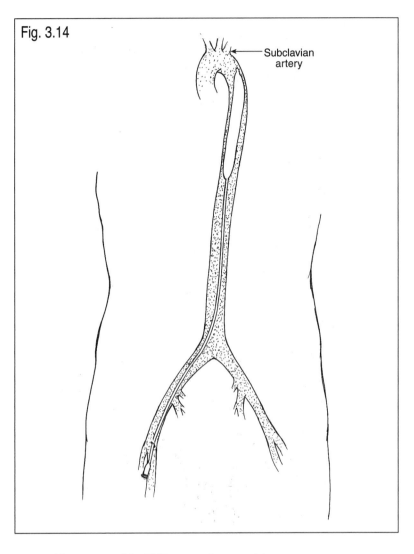

Fig. 3.14

Subclavian
artery

v. Obtain portable CXR to confirm position.
w. Initially, proper augmentation is accomplished with the
   IABP synchronized 1:2 with the patient's arterial pressure
   and then switched to a 1:1 augmentation.

7. Technique—Removal:
   a. Turn off IABP.
   b. Aspirate air from balloon to ensure deflation.
   c. Cut securing sutures and remove IABP catheter with a single
      swift pull.

d. Immediately place pressure over the insertion site with gauze pads in each hand. One hand is placed proximal to the entry site, and one distal.

e. Release pressure from the distal hand to allow a little back-bleeding from the distal vessel to dislodge any clot present (see Figure 3.15).

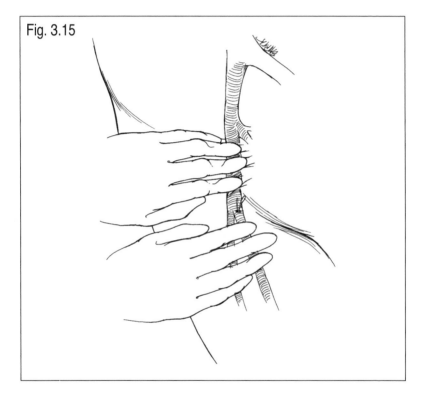

Fig. 3.15

f. Apply pressure with the distal hand and then release pressure from the proximal hand for 1–2 seconds, allowing forward bleeding to dislodge clots (see Figure 3.16).

g. Hold manual pressure for a minimum of 30 minutes (see Figure 3.17).

h. The patient should remain supine with legs extended for 6 hours with a pressure bag in place.

i. Make frequent checks of the groin area for hematoma formation.

j. Monitor distal pulses regularly.

Fig. 3.16

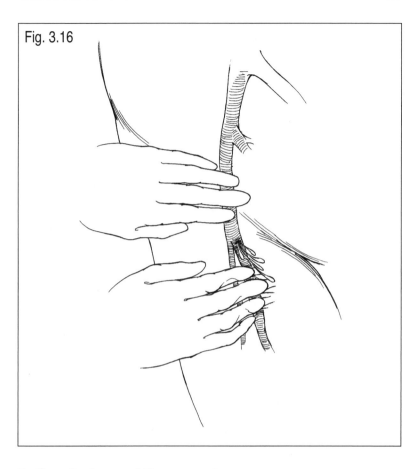

8. Complications and Management:

a. Limb ischemia of lower extremities
- Manifested by decreased or absent peripheral pulses, a pale or blue skin discoloration, a relative decrease in skin temperature of the affected extremity, extremity pain, or paresthesias.
- Document preinsertion and postinsertion pedal pulses. Assess the risk–benefit ratio of removing the IABP versus loss of limb. Further management may require femoral artery exploration and/or thrombectomy.

b. Aortic dissection
- Caused by an intimal tear and flap made in the aorta during balloon insertion.
- Manifested by a poor augmentation tracing, failure of the balloon to unwrap, hypotension, or back pain.

Fig. 3.17

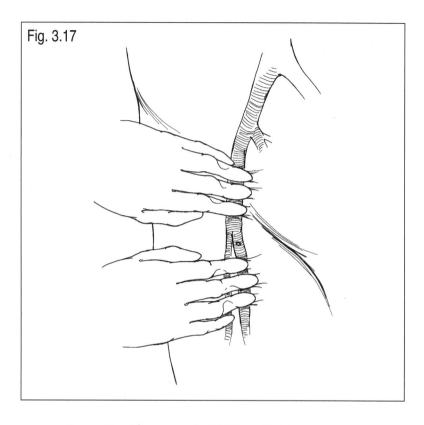

- Immediately remove the IABP and initiate appropriate surgical treatment.
c. Renal injury
  - Results either from thromboembolic events or secondary to occlusion of the orifice of the renal artery by the balloon.
  - Thrombectomy or proper repositioning of the balloon.
d. Thromboembolism
  - May lead to limb or organ ischemia and may be prevented with anticoagulation.
  - Embolectomy is sometimes successful.
e. Bleeding
  - Usually occurs at the insertion site, particularly if the patient is anticoagulated or has a coagulopathy.
  - Often readily controlled with local pressure.
f. Infection
  - Remove IABP.
  - Begin systemic antibiotics.

CHAPTER 4

THORACIC PROCEDURES

Authors: Herbert J. Zeh III, M.D. and
Kevin F. Staveley–O'Carroll, M.D.

THORACIC PROCEDURES

Bedside thoracic procedures may be diagnostic, therapeutic, or in certain situations, life-saving. All house officers should be familiar with the diagnosis and treatment of pleural effusion and pneumothorax. Also included in this section are recommendations for chemical pleural sclerosis and emergency bedside thoracotomy.

A. THORACENTESIS

1. Indications:
   a. Diagnostic thoracentesis is performed to determine the specific cause of a pleural effusion.
   b. Therapeutic thoracentesis is performed to relieve dyspnea

2. Contraindications:

   There are no absolute contraindications to thoracentesis; relative contraindications include the following:
   a. Coagulopathy (PT or PTT < 1.3 ratio, platelets < 50,000)
   b. Small-volume pleural fluid
   c. Mechanical ventilation
   d. Uncooperative patient

3. Anesthesia:

   1% lidocaine

4. Equipment:

   Several commercially available kits are available with a variety of silastic catheters and one-way valves. Manufacturers' instructions should be consulted for information unique to each system. If commercially available thoracentesis set is not available, a single-lumen central line kit may be used as described.

   a. Sterile prep solution
   b. Sterile gloves and towels
   c. 22- and 25-gauge needles
   d. 18-gauge insertion needle
   e. 16-gauge single-lumen central line and dilator
   f. 0.035-inch-diameter J wire
   g. Fine scissors
   h. Nonvented IV tubing
   i. Extension tubing
   j. Three-way stopcock
   k. 10 and 30 ml or larger syringe
   l. Vacuum bottles.

5. Positioning:

Sitting erect on the edge of the bed resting their head and extended arms on a bedside table (see Figure 4.1). Alternatively, in mechanically ventilated patients, thoracentesis may be performed in the lateral recumbent position.

6. Technique:

   a. Percuss the chest and identify the inferior margin and superior margin of the pleural effusion. Mark these landmarks on the patient's skin. If the lateral recumbent position is used or if the pleural effusion is small and/or loculated, ultrasound guidance should be used to accurately identify the safest site for thoracentesis.
   b. Prep and drape the area in the usual sterile fashion.
   c. Cut side holes in the 16-gauge catheter by folding it in half and cutting the edge of the fold with fine scissors. No more than one third of the catheter's diameter should be cut to avoid weakening the catheter and shearing on removal from the chest.
   d. Locate the rib two interspaces below the top of the effusion, but not below the eighth intercostal space. Raise a skin wheal with a 25-gauge needle and 1% lidocaine at that interspace, in the midscapular line. Alternatively, anesthetize a point two finger-breaths below the tip of the scapula.
   e. Using a 22-gauge needle, infiltrate the skin, subcutaneous tissue, and periosteum of the rib. Carefully walk the needle

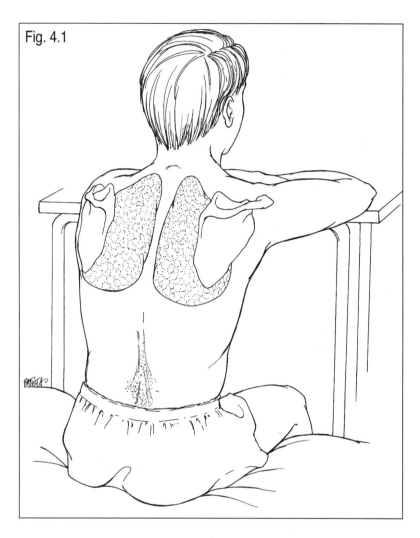

Fig. 4.1

superiorly over the edge of the rib while infiltrating with lidocaine. Once over the top of the rib, slowly advance the
needle while aspirating; until pleural fluid is encountered,
administer an additional 1–2 ml of lidocaine and then withdraw the needle (see Figure 4.2).
f. Place the 18-gauge needle on a 10-ml syringe, and insert it
into the pleural space as described above. It is often helpful
to use a two-handed technique with one hand stabilizing the
shaft of the needle at the skin surface and the other aspirating the syringe. This decreases the chances of the needle entering the lung if the patient inadvertently moves. Make sure

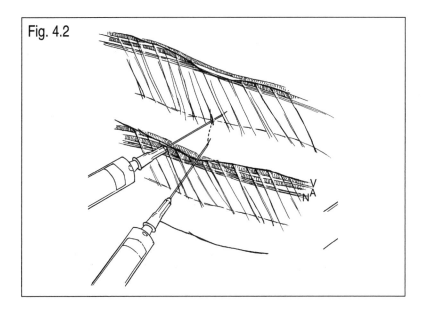

Fig. 4.2

that the bevel of the needle is directed inferiorly; this will ensure that the wire will pass inferiorly into the effusion (see Figure 4.3). Once pleural fluid is encountered, remove the syringe and place a finger over the needle to prevent air from entering the pleural cavity.

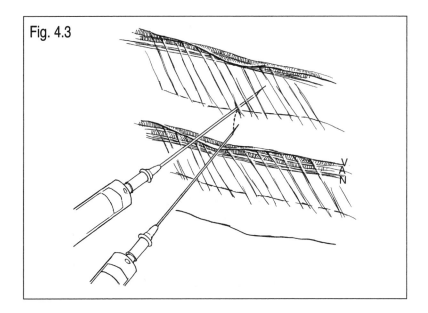

Fig. 4.3

g. Using the Seldinger technique, insert the wire through the needle into the chest, and then carefully remove the needle, leaving the wire (see Figure 4.4).

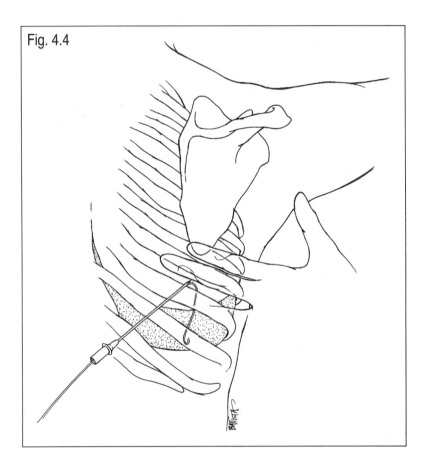

Fig. 4.4

h. With the scalpel, carefully make a small nick in the skin at the site of the wire insertion to allow easy introduction of the dilator.
i. Introduce the dilator over the wire to dilate the skin and sub-cutaneous tissues. The dilator should not be introduced any farther than is necessary to dilate the subcutaneous tissue and allow smoother insertion of the catheter.
j. Insert the catheter into the chest over the wire and then re-move the wire. Keep a finger over the end of the catheter to prevent air from entering the chest.

k. Connect the extension tubing and vacuum apparatus (see Figure 4.5).

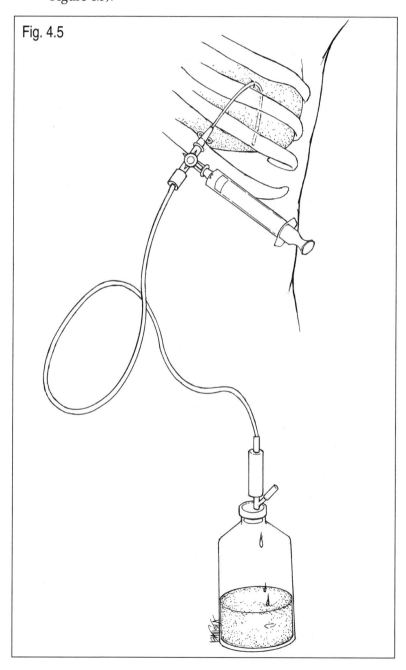

Fig. 4.5

l. Open the stopcock and withdraw fluid. Once the return of fluid has slowed, reposition the patient on the side and then the back to improve flow.

m. Slowly withdraw catheter to remove any pockets of fluid located proximal to the tip.

n. Place Betadine ointment and a dry sterile dressing on the puncture site. An occlusive dressing is generally not necessary because the needle tract will seal.

o. Obtain a CXR to rule out pneumothorax and evaluate remaining fluid.

7. **Complications and Management:**

a. Intercostal vessel damage
   - Risk of lacerating the intercostal vessels is minimized by positioning needle closely to the superior edge of the rib (see Figure 4.3).
   - If a laceration occurs, monitor hemodynamics closely and obtain serial CXRs. If the hemothorax is significant, tube thoracostomy may be necessary.

b. Poor flow
   - Rotate the patient in all directions to mobilize the thoracic fluid.
   - Occasionally manual aspiration of the fluid with a 30- to 60-ml syringe placed on a three-way stopcock may be useful.
   - Consider tube thoracostomy if effusion is viscous and unable to be drained adequately.

c. Pneumothorax—occurs through either lung puncture or leakage of exogenous air
   - Keep air out of the system at all times.
   - Stabilize the needle on insertion and do not advance needle after fluid is aspirated.
   - Monitor with serial CXRs. If the pneumothorax is significant or increasing (> 20%), tube thoracostomy.

B. TUBE THORACOSTOMY

Tube thoracostomy is performed to evacuate an ongoing production of air/fluid into the pleural space or fluid that is too viscous to be aspirated by thoracentesis. If there is any question of a tension pneumothorax, a 14-gauge or 16-gauge angiocatheter should immediately be placed in the second or third intercostal space in the midclavicular line on the ipsilateral side before a CXR and tube thoracostomy.

1. Indications:

    a. Posterior chest tube
- Hemothorax
- Pneumothorax (> 15%)
- Symptomatic pneumothorax of any size
- Persistent pleural effusion
- Empyema

    b. Anterior chest tube
- Pneumothorax (> 15%)

2. Contraindications:

None

3. Anesthesia:

1% lidocaine, IV sedation optional

4. Equipment:

    a. Sterile prep solution
    b. Sterile gloves and towels
    c. 3/4-inch 25-gauge needle
    d. 1 1/2-inch 22-gauge needle
    e. Chest tube #12 through #28F for pneumothoracies and #34F through #40F for fluid drainage
    f. 0 sutures on cutting needles (two)
    g. #15 blade
    h. Long Kelly clamps (two)
    i. Long tonsillar clamp
    j. 10- to 20- ml syringe
    k. Heavy scissors
    l. A Pleur-evac filled with sterile water according to the accompanying insert
    m. Xeroform gauze
    n. Sterile dressing
    o. Cloth tape
    p. Benzoin solution

5. Positioning:

Supine with the ipsilateral arm raised above the head to widen the intercostal space.

6. Technique—Posterior Approach:

   a. Identify the fifth intercostal space in the anterior axillary line—this is where the tube will enter the pleural space; the incision is made at the level of the sixth intercostal space lateral to the nipple but medial to the edge of the latissimus dorsi (see Figure 4.6).

   b. Sterile prep and drape the hemothorax.

   c. Raise a skin wheal with the 25-gauge needle, and with the 22-gauge needle infiltrate the entire area with 1% lidocaine. It is important to infiltrate at the level of the pleura and pos-

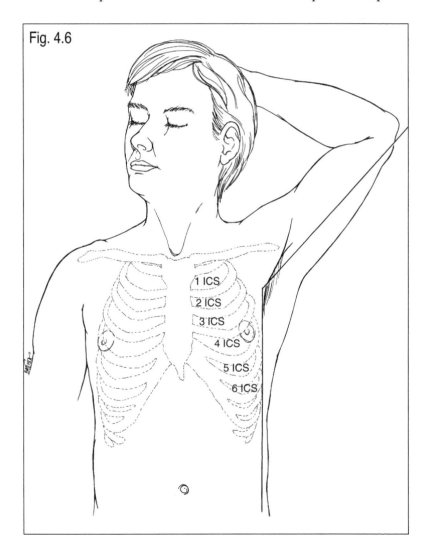

Fig. 4.6

1 ICS
2 ICS
3 ICS
4 ICS
5 ICS
6 ICS

terior periosteum. This level can be located by drawing back slightly after entering the pleural space with the 22-gauge finder needle.

d. Intercostal blocks may be administered for additional anesthesia by injecting 3–5 ml of lidocaine adjacent to the neurovascular bundle of the rib above and below the fifth intercostal space. Care should be taken to avoid injury to the intercostal artery and vein.

e. Make an incision through the skin parallel to the axis of the ribs. The length of the incision may vary but should be long enough to allow insertion of a finger and chest tube concurrently.

f. Measure the chest tube on the outside of the patient's body and identify how far the tube should be advanced after placement. The tip of the tube should be at the apex of the lung, about 8–12 cm from the last hole in the chest tube in a 70-kg adult (see Figure 4.7).

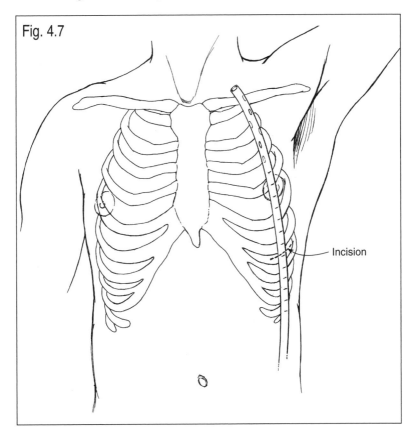

Fig. 4.7

Incision

g. With the tonsillar clamp, create a tract from the incision site to the intercostal space above (see Figure 4.8).

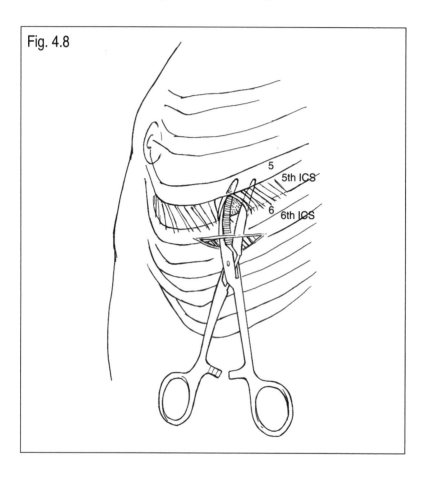

Fig. 4.8

5
5th ICS
6
6th ICS

h. Once the anterior intercostal fascia is identified, the tonsillar clamp is advanced into the pleural space by rolling the clamp over the superior edge of the rib to avoid injury to the neurovascular bundle.

i. On entering the pleural space, a rush of air should be heard. Do not advance the clamp any farther; dilate the tract with the clamp by spreading it widely. It is important to ensure that the tract is adequately dilated before removing the clamp; failure to do so often requires the reinsertion of the clamp and creation of a new tract into the pleural space.

j. Place a finger through the tract into the pleural space. Palpate the lung to confirm location in the pleural space and to ensure that no adhesions are present. A chest tube should never be inserted blindly because injury to the vessels or lung parenchyma may occur.

k. Place one Kelly clamp on the distal end of the chest tube.

l. Grasp the proximal end of the tube in the jaws of another Kelly clamp and insert both through the subcutaneous tract into the pleural cavity. Direct the tube posteriorly toward the apex (see Figure 4.9).

m. Open the jaws and remove the proximal Kelly clamp while advancing the tube to the predetermined position.

n. Alternatively you may insert and direct the tube by using a finger placed into the incision through the tract.

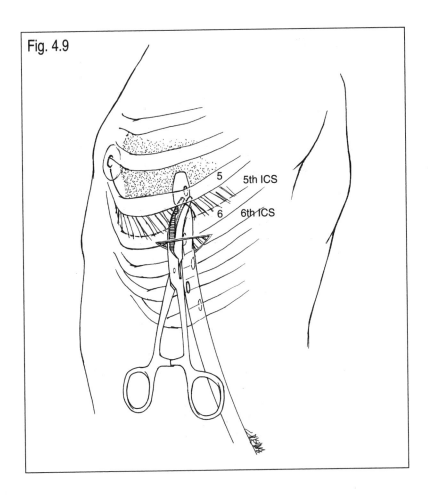

Fig. 4.9

5   5th ICS
6   6th ICS

o. Attach the tube to the Pleur-evac and remove the distal Kelly clamp.

p. To secure the chest tube: First place two large vertical mattress sutures on either side of the tube. Next reapproximate the skin incision, leaving long tails on each suture. Then wrap the remaining portion of each suture around the chest tube to secure it. When the chest tube is removed, only the portion of the suture attached to the chest tube should be cut, leaving the vertical mattress sutures in place to close the wound.

q. Place a piece of Xeroform gauze around the entrance site and a sterile dressing on top. Fasten securely with Benzoin and cloth tape.

r. Confirm placement with a CXR.

7. Technique—Anterior Approach:

a. Obtain a #24 tube or smaller.

b. Identify the second intercostal space lateral to the sternal angle of Louie in the midclavicular line.

c. Sterile prep and drape the hemothorax.

d. Raise a skin wheal with the 25-gauge needle, and with the 22-gauge needle infiltrate the entire area with 1% lidocaine. It is important to infiltrate at the level of the pleura and posterior periosteum. This level can be located by drawing back slightly after entering the pleural space with the 22-gauge finder needle.

e. Make an incision into the skin and carry it down through the subcutaneous tissue

f. Measure the chest tube on the outside of the patient's body to identify how far the tube should be advanced after placement.

g. With the tonsillar clamp, create a tract from the incision site superiorly, posteriorly, and immediately above the superior edge of the third rib to avoid injury to the neurovascular bundle (see Figure 4.10).

h. On entering the pleural space, a rush of air should be heard. Do not advance the clamp any farther; dilate the subcutaneous tract with the clamp by spreading it open.

i. Place a finger through the tract into the pleural space. Palpate the lung to confirm location in the pleural space and to ensure that no adhesions are present. A chest tube should never be inserted blindly because injury to the vessels or lung parenchyma may occur.

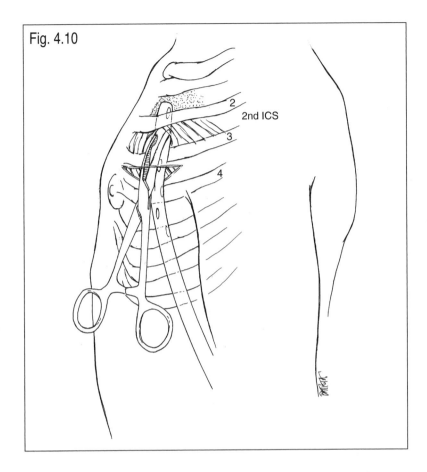

Fig. 4.10

2
2nd ICS
3
4

j. Place one Kelly clamp on the distal end of the chest tube.
k. Grasp the proximal end of the tube in the jaws of another Kelly clamp, and insert both through the subcutaneous tract into the pleural cavity. Direct the tube anteriorly toward the apex.
l. Open the jaws and remove the proximal Kelly clamp while advancing the tube to the predetermined position.
m. Attach the tube to the Pleur-evac and remove the distal Kelly clamp.
n. To secure the chest tube: First place two large vertical mattress sutures on either side of the tube. Next reapproximate the skin incision, leaving long tails on each suture. Then wrap the remaining portion of each suture around the chest tube to secure it. When the chest tube is removed, only the portion of the suture attached to the chest tube should be

cut, leaving the vertical mattress sutures in place to close the wound.

o. Place a piece of Xeroform gauze around the entrance site and a sterile dressing on top. Fasten securely with Benzoin and cloth tape.

p. Confirm placement with a CXR.

8. Technique—Chest Tube Removal:

a. Cut portion of the suture anchoring the tube, taking care not to cut the vertical mattress sutures that are reapproximating the skin.

b. Place Xeroform gauze and sterile gauze dressing over the insertion site.

c. While maintaining constant pressure on the skin with the gauze, ask the patient to take a deep breath and perform a Valsalva maneuver. Remove the tube during the Valsalva maneuver. This prevents air from entering the pleural cavity and causing a pneumothorax.

d. Have an assistant maintain the pressure seal on the skin while you tie the horizontal mattress suture, thereby closing the skin.

e. Place a dressing on top of the site. The sutures may be removed in 1 week.

f. Obtain a CXR to rule out a pneumothorax.

9. Complications and Management:

a. Poor positioning
   • The tube should be at the apex of the pleural cavity. It occasionally gets trapped in the major fissure of the lung.
   • Withdraw tube and re-insert. A second insertion site may be necessary if this is unsuccessful.

b. Persistent pneumothorax
   • Make sure all clamps are off the tubes and connection lines, and that there is not an obstruction in the system.
   • Check for an air leak in the system by clamping the tube at the chest wall. Air bubbling in the water seal chamber while on suction indicates a leak. Change the Pleur-evac system.
   • Repeat CXR in 4 hours. If still present, higher suction up to −40 cm can be achieved with an Emerson pump. If still no success, then a second tube should be placed via the anterior approach.

   c. Hemorrhage or lung injury
- Monitor hemodynamics and chest tube output, and obtain serial CXR.
- If output is > 200 ml/hr or 1.5 L total or patient is unstable, then emergent thoracotomy is indicated.

   d. Cardiac dysrhythmias
- Withdraw chest tube 1–3 cm if adjacent to heart. If it still persists, withdraw and re-insert via a new incision.
- Medical management if necessary

C. TROCAR CATHETER ("PIG-STICKER") THORACOSTOMY

1. Indications:

These catheters require minimal dissection and may be inserted quickly through a small incision. However, larger trocars can be difficult to place safely. For this reason we recommend that this technique be used only to place smaller tubes (12F or smaller) through an anterior approach. This can be very useful in treating smaller pneumothoracies, in which the risk of air leak is minimal.

2. Contraindications:

A standard chest tube should be placed rather than a trocar catheter in the following situations:
- Hemothorax
- Significant pneumothorax (> 15%)
- Persistent pleural effusion
- Empyema

3. Anesthesia:

1% lidocaine, IV sedation optional

4. Equipment:

   a. Sterile prep solution
   b. Sterile gloves and towels
   c. 3/4-inch 25-gauge needle
   d. 1 1/2-inch 22-gauge needle
   e. 60-ml syringe
   f. Argyle Trocar catheter 20F to 24F
   g. 0 sutures on cutting needles (two)

  h. #15 blade and scalpel handle
  i. Kelly clamp
  j. Heavy scissors
  k. Pleur-evac filled with sterile water according to the insert
  l. Xeroform gauze
  m. Sterile dressing
  n. Cloth tape
  o. Benzoin solution

5. Positioning:

  Supine with the ipsilateral arm raised above the head to widen the intercostal space.

6. Technique:

  a. Identify the second intercostal space in the midclavicular line (see Figure 4.11).
  b. Sterile prep and drape the hemothorax.
  c. Raise a skin wheal with the 25-gauge needle, and with the 22-gauge needle infiltrate the entire area with 1% lidocaine. It is most important to infiltrate at the level of the pleural and posterior periosteum. This level can be located by drawing back slightly after entering the pleural space and obtaining air return with the 22-gauge finder needle.
  d. Measure the chest tube on the outside of the patient's body and identify how far the tube should be advanced after placement.
  e. Make a horizontal incision approximately 0.5–1.0 cm.
  f. Grasp the base of the trocar portion of trocar catheter in the palm of the right hand (see Figure 4.12). This hand will supply the driving force for the insertion. The trocar should be fully advanced within the catheter.
  g. Grasp the tip of the trocar catheter with the left hand and insert the unit through the incision.
  h. Using the left hand as a guide and apply gentle force with the right hand onto the trocar to tunnel the trocar catheter under the skin over the superior edge of the third rib, avoiding injury to the neurovascular bundle.
  i. Gently advance the entire unit not more than 2–3 cm into the pleural cavity, aiming for the apex. Too much force or excessive advancement can result in lung injury.
  j. Advance the catheter only over the trocar (hold the trocar

Fig. 4.11

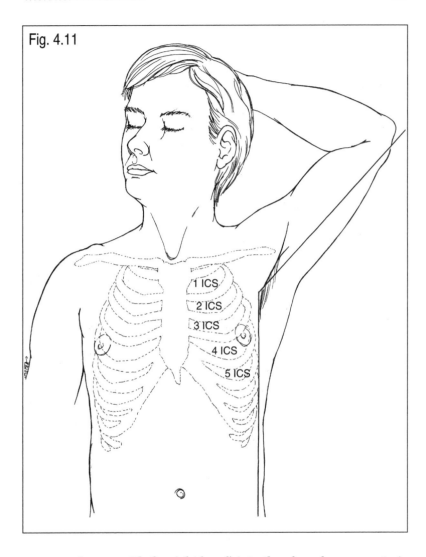

1 ICS
2 ICS
3 ICS
4 ICS
5 ICS

stationary with the right hand) into the pleural space posteriorly toward the apex to the desired length (see Figure 4.13).

k. Withdraw the trocar and clamp the end with a Kelly clamp.

l. Attach the tube to the Pleur-evac and remove the Kelly
clamp.

m. To secure the chest tube: First place two large vertical mattress sutures on either side of the tube. Next reapproximate
the skin incision, leaving long tails on each suture. Then
wrap the remaining portion of each suture around the chest
tube to secure it. When the chest tube is removed, only the

Fig. 4.12

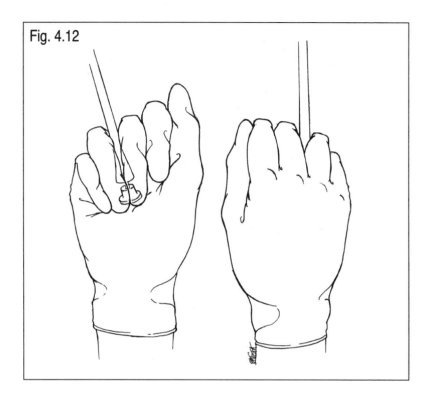

portion of the suture attached to the chest tube should be
cut, leaving the vertical mattress sutures in place to close the
wound.
n. Place a piece of Xeroform gauze around the entrance site and
a sterile dressing on top. Fasten securely with Benzoin and
cloth tape.
o. Confirm placement with a CXR.

7. Complications and Management:
    a. Poor positioning
        • The tube should be at the apex of the pleural cavity. It
          occasionally gets trapped in the major fissure of the lung. If
          this occurs, the tube should be removed and re-inserted.
          Frequently a separate insertion site is required to prevent
          recurrence.
    b. Persistent pneumothorax
        • Make sure all clamps are off the tubes and connection
          lines, and that there is not an obstruction in the system.

- Check for an air leak in the system by clamping the tube at the chest wall. Air bubbling in the water seal chamber indicates a leak. Change the Pleur-evac system.
- Repeat CXR in 4 hours. If still present, higher suction up to −60 cm can be achieved with an Emerson pump. If still no success, then a standard posterior tube thoracotomy should be performed.

c. Hemorrhage or lung injury
   - Monitor chest tube output and obtain serial CXR every 2 hours.

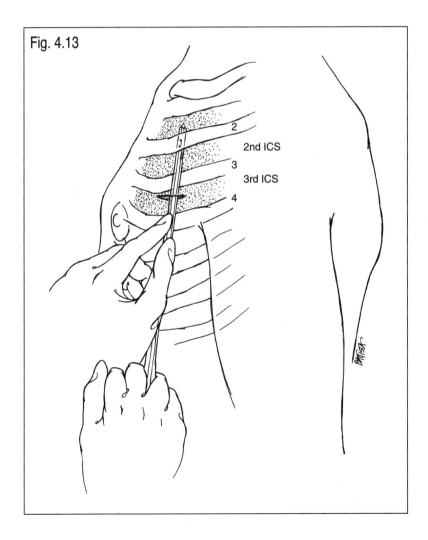

Fig. 4.13

- If hemodynamically unstable or if output is > 300 ml/hr or 2 L total, operative explanation is required.
  d. Cardiac dysrhythmias
    - Withdraw chest tube 1–3 cm if adjacent to heart. If still persists, withdraw and re-insert via a separate skin site.
    - Medical management if necessary

D. TECHNIQUE—PERCUTANEOUS (WIRE-DIRECTED) TUBE THORACOSTOMY

Several commercially available percutaneous tube thorascopy kits are available. Manufacturer's instructions should be consulted for information unique to each system.

1. Indications:

This can be very useful in treating smaller pneumothoracies, where the risk of air leak is minimal.

2. Contraindications:

A standard chest tube should be placed rather than a percutaneous catheter in the following situations:
- Hemothorax
- Significant pneumothorax (> 15%)
- Persistent pleural effusion
- Empyema

3. Anesthesia:

1% lidocaine, IV sedation optional

4. Equipment:

a. Sterile prep solution
b. Sterile gloves and towels
c. 3/4-inch 25-gauge needle
d. 18-gauge introducer needle
e. 0.38-inch diameter stainless steel J-tip wire
f. 20-ml syringe
g. Two sequentially larger dilators
h. Thal-quick chest tube with inserter trocar or other commercially available system
i. Two 0 vicryl sutures on cutting needles
j. #15 blade and scalpel handle

5. Positioning:

Supine with the ipsilateral arm raised above the head

6. Technique:

a. Prep and drape the hemithoraces in standard fashion.

b. Identify the fifth and sixth intercostal space in the midaxillary line.

c. Raise a skin wheal with the 25-gauge needle, and with the
   22-gauge needle infiltrate the entire area with 1% lidocaine.
   It is important to infiltrate at the level of the pleura and posterior periosteum. This level can be located by drawing back
   slightly after entering the pleural space with the 22-gauge
   finder needle.

d. Make a small incision slightly larger than the diameter of the
   chest tube.

e. Place the 18-gauge introducer needle on the syringe and insert into the incision. Direct the needle superiorly with the
   bevel directed up, and advance over the superior border of
   the rib while aspirating. Fluid or air should be aspirated to
   verify intrapleural position (see Figure 4.14).

f. Remove the syringe and advance the soft J end of the wire

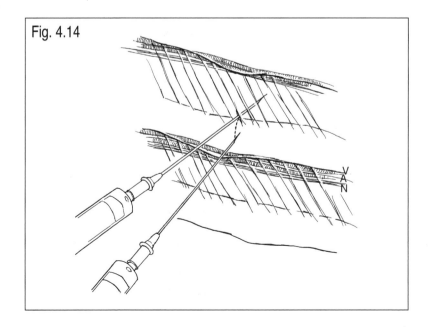

Fig. 4.14

through the needle and into the pleural space. The wire should advance without resistance (see Figure 4.15).

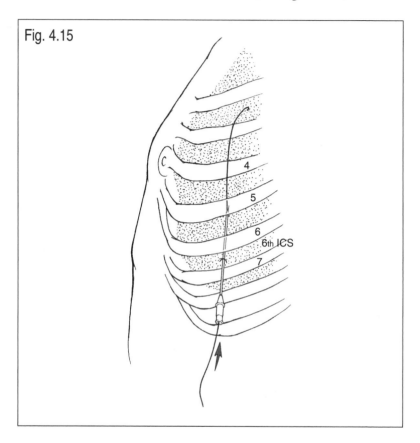

Fig. 4.15

g. Remove needle and leave wire in place.
h. While maintaining wire in position, sequentially dilate (smaller to larger) the tract by inserting the dilators over the wire. Introduction of the dilators may be facilitated by twisting and advancing in the same plane as the wire. The wire should freely move through the dilators at all times to prevent kinking of the wire. Dilators should never be advanced farther than the distance of the subcutaneous tract to avoid injury to the lung.
i. Insert the chest tube/inserter assembly over the wire into the pleural space to the premeasured length (see Figure 4.16).
j. Remove the wire and chest tube inserter trocar, leaving the chest tube in place.

Fig. 4.16

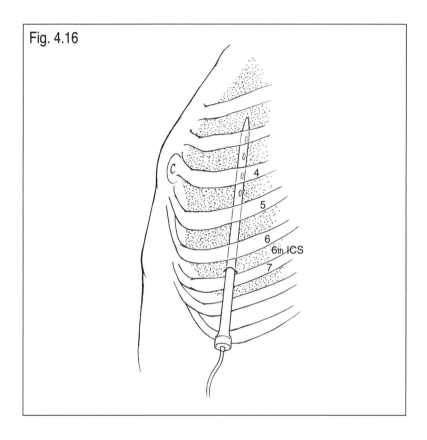

k. Attach the tube to the Pleur-evac.
l. To secure the chest tube: First place two large vertical mattress sutures on either side of the tube. Next reapproximate
   the skin incision, leaving long tails on each suture. Then wrap
   the remaining portion of each suture around the chest tube to
   secure it. When the chest tube is removed, only the portion of
   the suture attached to the chest tube should be cut, leaving
   the vertical mattress sutures in place to close the wound.
m. Place a piece of Xeroform gauze around the entrance site and
   a sterile dressing on top. Fasten securely with Benzoin and
   cloth tape.
n. Confirm placement with a CXR.

7. Complications and Management:
   a. Poor positioning
      • The tube should be at the apex of the pleural cavity. It

occasionally gets trapped in the major fissure of the lung. If this occurs, the tube should be removed and re-inserted. Frequently a separate insertion site is required to prevent recurrence.

b. Persistent pneumothorax
- Make sure all clamps are off the tubes and connection lines, and that there is not an obstruction in the system.
- Check for an air leak in the system by clamping the tube at the chest wall. Air bubbling in the water seal chamber indicates a leak. Change the Pleur-evac system.
- Repeat CXR in 4 hours. If still present, higher suction up to −60 cm can be achieved with an Emerson pump. If still no success, then a standard posterior tube thoracotomy should be performed.

c. Hemorrhage or lung injury
- Monitor chest tube output and obtain serial CXR every 2 hours.
- If hemodynamically unstable or if output is > 250 ml/hr or 1.5 L total, operative explanation is required.

d. Cardiac dysrhythmias
- Withdraw chest tube 1–3 cm if adjacent to heart. If still persists, withdraw and re-insert via a separate skin site.
- Medical management if necessary

E. CHEMICAL PLEURAL SCLEROSIS

Chemical pleural sclerosis is a bedside procedure used to obliterate the pleural space by inducing inflammation. A variety of substances have been used for pleural sclerosis. Currently the two most popular are talc and doxycycline. Talc pleural sclerosis has been shown to result in a lower recurrence rate of spontaneous pneumothorax than doxycycline. Also, talc is generally less painful to the patient than doxycycline.

1. Indications:
   a. Persistent pneumothorax (persistent air leak with the lung expanded)
   b. Recurrent malignant pleural effusions
   c. Recurrent spontaneous pneumothoracies (relative)
   d. Primary spontaneous pneumothorax (controversial)

2. Contraindications:
   Allergies to tetracycline, doxycycline, or talc

3. Anesthesia:

1% lidocaine (50 ml)

4. Equipment:

a. Kelly clamp
b. Sterile prep solution
c. Gauze
d. Sterile normal saline
e. Doxycycline or talc
f. 60-ml syringes (two)

5. Positioning:

Supine initially. Patient must have a chest tube and Pleur-evac in place.

6. Technique-Doxycycline:

a. Obtain doxycycline 500 mg in 50 ml normal saline and 40 ml of 1% lidocaine in two separate 60-ml syringes. Alternatively, the lidocaine and doxycycline may be admixed in a 1:1 mixture and instilled together.
b. Clamp the chest tube with a Kelly clamp near the entrance site at the skin.
c. Sterile prep the distal portion of the chest tube at the connection with the Pleur-evac tubing, and then disconnect the chest tube from the Pleur-evac.
d. Attach the 60-ml syringe containing the lidocaine to the end of the chest tube.
e. Remove the Kelly clamp, instill the lidocaine through the chest tube into the pleural cavity, and reclamp the chest tube.
f. Rotate the patient from side to side every 2 minutes for 10–15 minutes to distribute the lidocaine for anesthesia.
g. Fill the other 60-ml syringe with the doxycycline solution.
h. Attach the doxycycline syringe to the chest tube, remove the Kelly clamp, and instill the solution into the pleural cavity. Clamp the chest tube.
i. Repeat Steps g and h until 300–400 ml of doxycycline have been administered.
j. Rotate the patient to each of the following four positions every 30 minutes:
   • Left lateral decubitus
   • Right lateral decubitus

- Trendelenburg
- Reverse Trendelenburg

k. After 4 hours, replace the chest tube back to Pleur-evac suction for at least the next 24 hours, until the lung has fully expanded and no air leak is present.

7. Technique—Talc:

a. Obtain talc 5 g suspended in 250 ml normal saline and 40 ml of 1% lidocaine in two separate 60-ml syringes.

b. Clamp the chest tube with a Kelly clamp near the entrance site at the skin.

c. Sterile prep the distal portion of the chest tube at the connection with the Pleur-evac tubing, and then disconnect the patient's chest tube from the Pleur-evac.

d. Attach the 60-ml syringe containing the lidocaine to the end of the chest tube.

e. Remove the Kelly clamp, instill the lidocaine through the chest tube into the pleural cavity, and reclamp the chest tube.

f. Rotate the patient from side to side every 2 minutes for 10–15 minutes to distribute the lidocaine for anesthesia.

g. Fill the other 60-ml syringe with the talc solution.

h. Attach the talc syringe to the chest tube, remove the Kelly clamp, and instill the solution into the pleural cavity. Clamp the chest tube.

i. Repeat Steps g and h until all 250 ml of talc have been administered.

j. Rotate the patient to each of the following four positions every 30 minutes:
- Left lateral decubitus
- Right lateral decubitus
- Trendelenburg
- Reverse Trendelenburg

k. After 4 hours, replace the chest tube back to Pleur-evac suction for at least the next 24 hours, until the lung has fully expanded and no air leak is present.

F. EMERGENCY BEDSIDE THORACOTOMY

1. Indications:

Cardiac arrest in victims of penetrating trauma to the thorax who had vital signs in the field or on arrival to the emergency department. In certain situations emergency thoracotomy may be indicated in other penetrating trauma injuries.

2. Contraindications:

Emergency thoracotomy has not been shown to be effective in traumatic cardiac arrest secondary to blunt trauma.

3. Anesthesia:

None

4. Equipment:
a. Sterile prep solution
b. Sterile gloves and towels
c. #10 blade and scalpel handle
d. Chest wall retractor
e. Mayo scissors
f. Metzenbaum scissors
g. Smooth forceps
h. Toothed forceps
i. Aortic clamp
j. Suction apparatus

5. Positioning:

Supine

6. Technique:
a. Make an incision at the level of the left fifth intercostal space in the midclavicular line from sternum laterally as far as possible. With the scalpel, carry the incision down to bone directly over the fifth rib (see Figure 4.17).
b. Insert partially opened Mayo scissors over the superior aspect of the fifth rib (to avoid laceration of intercostal vessels) and open pleural space the entire length of the incision.
c. Insert the chest wall (rib spreader) retractor.
d. Elevate the left lung to expose the descending thoracic aorta (see Figure 4.18).
e. Bluntly dissect the mid-descending thoracic aorta circumferentially free from the posterior mediastinum and place an aortic clamp on it, being careful not to injure the esophagus anteriorly. A nasogastric tube (Chapter 5) can be placed to

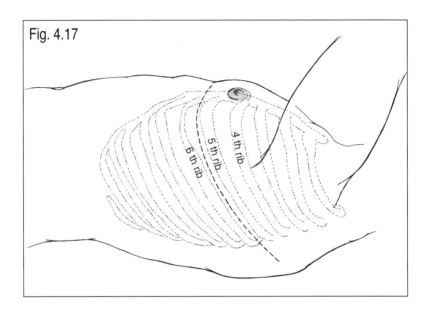

Fig. 4.17

4 th rib
5 th rib
6 th rib

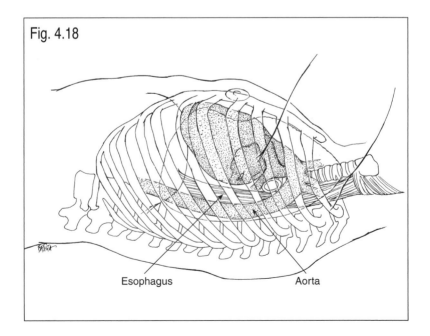

Fig. 4.18

Esophagus   Aorta

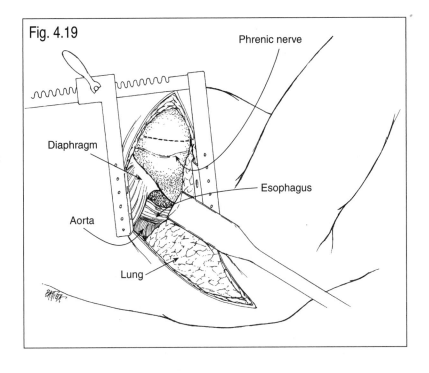

Fig. 4.19

Phrenic nerve

Diaphragm

Esophagus

Aorta

Lung

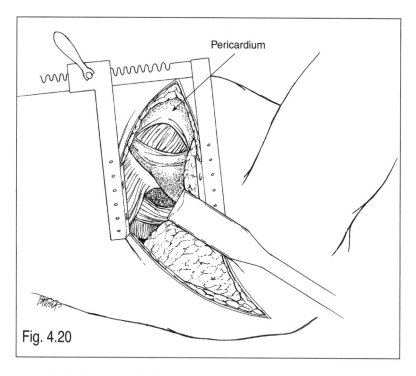

Fig. 4.20

help distinguish the esophagus from the aorta on palpation (see Figure 4.19).

f. Place aortic clamp across the aorta after it is mobilized.

g. Retract the left lung inferiorly and identify the pericardial sac.

h. Open the pericardial sac its entire length longitudinally (a longitudinal incision will prevent injury to the phrenic nerve).

i. Evacuate any clot in the pericardium, and deliver the heart into the left hemithorax for examination (see Figure 4.20).

j. Injuries to the heart may be quickly repaired at this time using pledgeted nonabsorbable (Prolene) suture.

k. Take the patient immediately to the operating room.

7. Complications and Management:

a. Internal mammary artery laceration
   • When lacerated, should be repaired in the operating room.

b. Poor exposure
   • Make the incision as wide as is practical considering the patient's supine position.

CHAPTER 5

GASTROINTESTINAL PROCEDURES

Robert C. Moesinger, M.D.

GASTROINTESTINAL PROCEDURES

Disorders of the abdomen are, in many ways, the essence of general surgery. The surgeon should have expertise in the anatomy of the abdomen and confidence in examination of the abdomen. Similarly, gastrointestinal procedures should be an integral part of the armamentarium of the general surgeon.

I. UPPER GASTROINTESTINAL PROCEDURES

Indications for intubation of the upper gastrointestinal (GI) tract include evacuation of the stomach (and occasionally more distal gastrointestinal tract) of gases and fluids for diagnostic and/or therapeutic purposes, or to deliver nutrients and medications. Modern GI tubes have a rich history; they are the product of many years of modifications in material and design.

A. NASOGASTRIC TUBES

1. Indications:
   a. Acute gastric dilatation
   b. Gastric outlet obstruction
   c. Upper gastrointestinal bleeding
   d. Ileus
   e. Small bowel obstruction
   f. Enteral feeding

2. Contraindications:
   a. Recent esophageal or gastric surgery
   b. Head trauma with possible basilar skull fracture

3. Anesthesia:

   None or viscous lidocaine in the nose

4. Equipment:
   a. Levin or Salem sump tube
   b. Water-soluble lubricant
   c. Catheter-tip syringe (60 ml)
   d. Cup of ice
   e. Stethoscope
   f. Cup of water with a straw

5. Positioning:

   Sitting or supine

6. Technique:
   a. Measure tube from mouth to earlobe and down to anterior abdomen so that last hole on tube is below the xiphoid process. This marks the distance that the tube should be inserted.
   b. Some surgeons will place tip of tube in cup of ice to stiffen it or bend the tip downward to facilitate the tube's passage into the proximal esophagus.
   c. Apply lubricant liberally to tube.
   d. Ask patient to flex neck, and gently insert tube into a patent naris (see Figure 5.1).
   e. Advance tube into nasopharynx aiming posteriorly, asking the patient to swallow if possible.
   f. Once the tube has been swallowed, confirm that the patient can speak clearly and breathe without difficulty, and gently advance tube to estimated length. If the patient is able, instruct him or her to drink water through a straw; while the patient swallows, gently advance the tube.
   g. Confirm correct placement into the stomach by injecting approximately 20 ml of air with catheter-tip syringe while auscultating epigastric area. Return of a large volume of fluid through tube also confirms placement into stomach.

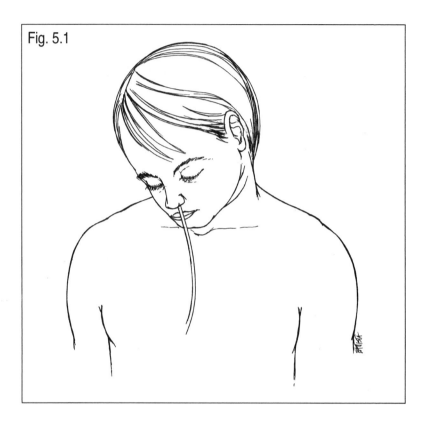

Fig. 5.1

h. Carefully tape tube to the patient's nose, ensuring that pressure is not applied by tube against naris. Tube should be kept well lubricated to prevent erosion at naris. With the use of tape and a safety pin, the tube can be secured to the patient's gown.
 i. Irrigate tube with 30 ml of normal saline every 4 hours. Salem sump tubes will also require the injection of 30 ml of air through the sump (blue) port every 4 hours to maintain proper functioning.
 j. Constant low suction may be applied to Salem sump tubes, whereas Levin tubes should have only low intermittent suction.
 k. Monitor gastric pH every 4–6 hours and correct with antacids for pH < 4.5.
 l. Monitor gastric residuals if tube is used for enteral feeding. Obtain a chest radiograph to confirm correct placement before using any tube for enteral feeding.
m. The tube ideally should not be clamped because it stents

open the lower esophagus, increasing the risk of aspiration if the patient's stomach should distend.

7. Complications and Management:

a. Pharyngeal discomfort
  • Common due to the large caliber of these tubes.
  • Throat lozenges or sips of water may provide relief.
  • Avoid using aerosolized anesthetic for the pharynx because this may inhibit the gag reflex, interfering with the protective mechanism of the airway.
b. Erosion of the naris
  • Prevented by keeping tube well lubricated and ensuring that tube is taped so that pressure is not applied against naris. Tube should always be lower than the nose and never taped to the forehead of the patient.
  • Frequent checking of the tube position at the naris can help prevent this problem.
c. Sinusitis
  • Occurs with long-term use of nasogastric tubes.
  • Remove the tube and place in other naris.
  • Antibiotic therapy if needed.
d. Nasotracheal intubation
  • Results in airway obstruction that is fairly easy to diagnose in the awake patient (cough, inability to speak).
  • Obtain a chest radiograph to confirm placement prior to use for enteral feeding.
e. Gastritis
  • Usually manifests itself as mild, self-limited upper gastrointestinal bleeding.
  • Prophylaxis consists of maintaining gastric pH > 4.5 with antacids via the tube, intravenous (IV) histamine$_2$ receptor blockers, and removal of tube as soon as possible.
f. Epistaxis
  • Usually self-limited.
  • If persists, remove the tube and assess location of bleed.
  • Refer to Chapter 1 for treatment of anterior and posterior epistaxis.

B. OROGASTRIC TUBE

1. Indications:

The indications for orogastric (OG) tubes are generally the same as for NG tubes. However, because they are generally not tolerated well by the awake patient, they are used in intubated patients and newborns. The OG tube is the preferred tube for decompressing the stomach in the head trauma patient with a potential basilar skull fracture.

    a. Acute gastric dilatation
    b. Gastric outlet obstruction
    c. Upper gastrointestinal bleeding
    d. Ileus
    e. Small bowel obstruction
    f. Enteral feeding

2. Contraindications:

Recent esophageal or gastric surgery

3. Anesthesia:

None

4. Equipment:

    a. Levin or Salem sump tube
    b. Water-soluble lubricant
    c. Catheter-tip syringe (60 ml)
    d. Stethoscope

5. Positioning:

Supine

6. Technique:

    a. Measure tube from mouth to earlobe and down to anterior abdomen so that last hole on tube is below the xiphoid process. This marks the distance the tube should be inserted.
    b. Apply lubricant liberally to tube.
    c. Because the patients in whom OG tubes are used are generally unable to cooperate, the tube should be placed into the mouth, directed posteriorly, until the tip begins to pass downward into the esophagus.
    d. Advance the tube slowly and steadily. If any resistance is encountered, stop and withdraw the tube completely. Repeat step c.
    e. If the tube advances easily, with little resistance, continue until the premeasured distance is reached. Resistance, gag-

ging, fogging of the tube, or hypoxia suggests errant placement of the tube into the trachea.

f. Confirm correct placement into stomach by injecting 20 ml of air with the catheter-tip syringe while auscultating over the epigastric area. Correct placement is also confirmed by aspiration of a large volume of fluid.

g. Irrigate tube with 15–20 ml of saline every 4 hours. Salem sump tubes will require injection of 15–20 ml of air through the sump (blue) port every 4 hours to maintain proper functioning.

h. Constant low suction may be applied to Salem sump tubes, whereas Levin tubes should have only low intermittent suction.

i. Monitor gastric residuals if tube is used for enteral feeding. Obtain a chest radiograph to confirm placement before using for enteral feeding.

j. Monitor gastric pH every 4–6 hours and correct with antacids for pH < 4.5.

7. Complications and Management:

a. Pharyngeal discomfort and gagging are a problem with OG tubes when they are placed in awake and alert patients, and essentially eliminates their use in such patients except in conjunction with an oral endotracheal tube.

b. Tracheal intubation
- Correct placement in the esophagus is usually evident by the ease of advancement of the tube. Any resistance suggests tracheal intubation or coiling within the posterior pharynx.
- Obtain a chest radiograph to confirm placement prior to use for enteral feeding.

c. Gastritis
- Usually manifests itself as mild, self-limited upper gastrointestinal bleeding.
- Prophylaxis consists of maintaining gastric pH > 4.5 with antacids via the tube, IV histamine$_2$ receptor blockers, and removal of tube as soon as possible.

C. NASODUODENAL TUBE

1. Indications:

Enteral feeding

2. Contraindications:

Recent esophageal or gastric surgery

3. Anesthesia:

None or viscous lidocaine in the nose

4. Equipment:

   a. Tip-weighted, small-caliber tube
   b. Guide wire
   c. Water-soluble lubricant
   d. Cup of water with a straw
   e. Stethoscope
   f. Catheter-tip syringe

5. Positioning:

Sitting or supine

6. Technique:

   a. Measure tube length from mouth to earlobe and down to
      anterior abdomen so that tip is 6 cm below xiphoid
      process.
   b. Most duodenal tube tips are self-lubricating when moistened
      with water. If not, apply water-soluble lubricant to the tip of
      the tube.
   c. Ask patient to flex neck, and gently insert the tube contain-
      ing the guide wire into a patent naris.
   d. Advance tube into pharynx aiming posteriorly, asking the
      patient to swallow if possible.
   e. Once the tube has been swallowed, confirm that the patient
      can speak clearly and breathe without difficulty, and gently
      advance tube to estimated length. If the patient is able, in-
      struct him or her to drink water through a straw, and while
      the patient swallows, gently advance the tube.
   f. Confirm correct placement into stomach by injecting approx-
      imately 20 ml of air with catheter-tip syringe while auscultat-
      ing the epigastric area.
   g. Remove the guide wire and ask the patient to lie in a right
      decubitus position for 1–2 hours. An abdominal radiograph
      at this point will confirm transpyloric tube position or that
      the tube is coiled in the stomach; if coiled, withdraw tube for

some distance and repeat this step. The tube should not be fixed to the nose.

h. The patient should first lie in a supine position for 1–2 hours and then in a left decubitus position for 1–2 hours to facilitate passage of the tube through the C-loop of the duodenum.

i. At this point, position of the tube should be confirmed by radiograph. If the tube has not passed beyond the stomach by this time, then upper endoscopy or fluoroscopy may be necessary to advance the tube into the duodenum.

7. Complications and Management:

a. Epistaxis
- Usually self-limited.
- If persistent, remove the tube and assess location of bleed.
- Refer to Chapter 1 for treatment of anterior and posterior epistaxis.

b. Intestinal perforation
- Presents usually as free air on chest radiograph.
- Caused by inserting guide wire back through lumen of tube while it is in place. This should never be done.

c. Obstruction of lumen (see section F below)

D. LONG INTESTINAL TUBE

1. Indications:

Early partial small bowel obstruction

2. Contraindications:

a. Uncooperative patient
b. Indication for operative intervention (i.e., small bowel ischemia)

3. Anesthesia:

None or viscous lidocaine in the nose

4. Equipment:

a. Long intestinal tube
b. Water-soluble lubricant

  c. Saline
  d. 5-ml syringe, 22-gauge needle

5. Positioning:

  Sitting up initially, then variable position as described below

6. Technique:

  a. Using needle and syringe, inject 5 ml of saline into the bal-
     loon at the end of the tube (see Figure 5.2).
  b. With the patient in an upright sitting position, roll up the
     balloon, apply a liberal amount of lubricant, and insert bal-
     loon into a patent naris.
  c. Carefully manipulate the tube such that the balloon falls into
     the nasopharynx without obstructing the airway.
  d. Instruct the patient to swallow the balloon as it is lowered
     slowly into the pharynx as though it were a bolus of food.
     Passage of the balloon in the patient who cannot swallow
     may be difficult. Often the balloon will advance along with
     the tube.
  e. After balloon has been swallowed, confirm that the patient
     can speak clearly and breathe easily, then advance it slowly

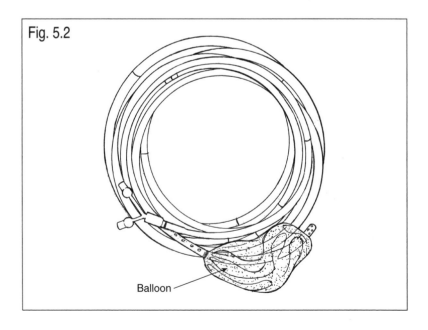

Fig. 5.2

Balloon

into the stomach by instructing the patient to continue swallowing.

f. Insert the tube to the point at which the D mark is at the nose, and have the patient lie in a right decubitus position for 1–2 hours. The tube should not be fixed to the nose. Low intermittent suction may be applied.

g. Obtain an abdominal radiograph to confirm the presence of the tip in the duodenum or that the tube is coiled in the stomach and may need to be withdrawn for some distance.

h. The patient should then be placed supine for 1–2 hours, then next in a left decubitus position for 1–2 additional hours to facilitate passage of the tube through the C-loop of the duodenum.

i. At this point, position of the tube should be confirmed again by abdominal radiograph. If the tube has not passed beyond the stomach by this time, placement of the tip through the pylorus by flexible upper endoscopy or under fluoroscopy may be necessary.

j. Once the tube is in the duodenum, it can be advanced 2–3 cm every 15 minutes.

k. Once the tube is no longer needed, removal should proceed slowly over several hours to prevent intussusception (withdraw tube 3–5 cm every 10–15 minutes).

7. Complications and Management:

a. Airway obstruction
   • The balloon may occlude the upper airway during initial placement.
   • Withdraw the tube immediately.

b. Epistaxis
   • Usually self-limited.
   • If it persists, remove the tube and assess location of bleed.
   • Refer to Chapter 1 for treatment of anterior and posterior epistaxis.

c. Intussusception of small intestine during removal
   • Best avoided by withdrawing tube 3–5 cm every 10–15 minutes.

E. SENGSTAKEN-BLAKEMORE TUBE

The Sengstaken-Blakemore (SB) tube is an emergently placed tube that temporarily stops life-threatening hemorrhage from gastroesophageal varices. It is only a temporizing therapy before definitive operative, endoscopic, or transjugular intrahepatic portosystemic shunt procedure.

1. Indications:

   Exsanguinating hemorrhage from gastroesophageal varices

2. Contraindications:

   None

3. Anesthesia:

   None or viscous lidocaine in the nose

4. Equipment:

   a. SB tube
   b. Catheter-tip 60-ml syringe
   c. Hemostat clamps (two)
   d. Pressure manometer
   e. Levine or Salem sump NG tube
   f. Water-soluble lubricant
   g. Scissors

5. Positioning:

   Supine or lateral decubitus

6. Technique:

   a. Because potentially lethal complications can occur with the use of the SB tube, patients should be in a monitored setting, such as the intensive care unit, staffed by personnel experienced with the use of this device.
   b. Control of the airway by endotracheal intubation is strongly advised to minimize the risk of aspiration.
   c. Pass a large NG tube (see section I A) or OG tube (see section I B) to empty the stomach of blood, and then remove the tube.
   d. Inflate both esophageal and gastric balloons of the SB tube with air to test for leaks, then deflate.
   e. Apply lubricant liberally to the tube.
   f. Ask patient to flex neck, and gently insert tube into a patent naris.

g. Advance tube into pharynx, aiming posteriorly and asking the patient to swallow if possible.

h. Once the tube has been swallowed, confirm that the patient can speak clearly and breathe without difficulty (if not intubated), and gently advance tube to approximately 45 cm.

i. Apply low intermittent suction to the gastric aspiration port. Return of blood should confirm placement in the stomach. Otherwise inject 20 ml of air with the catheter-tip syringe while auscultating epigastric area (see Figure 5.3).

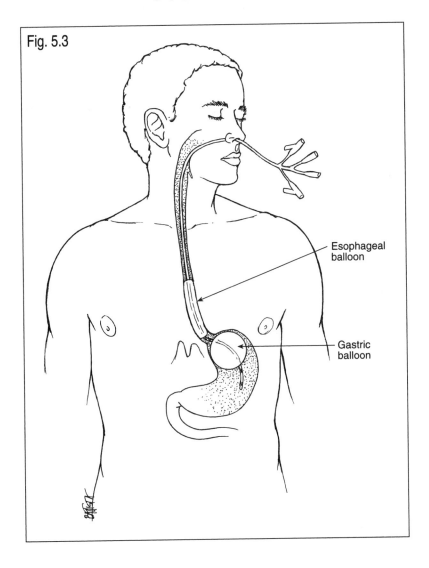

Fig. 5.3

Esophageal balloon

Gastric balloon

j. Slowly inject 100 ml of air into the gastric balloon and then clamp the balloon port to prevent air leakage. Stop inflating the balloon immediately if the patient complains of pain because this could indicate that the balloon is in the esophagus. If this is the case, deflate the gastric balloon, advance the tube an additional 10 cm, and repeat the injection of air.

k. With the gastric balloon inflated, slowly withdraw the tube until resistance is met at the gastroesophageal junction. Anchor the tube to the patient's nose under minimal tension with padding.

l. Obtain a chest radiograph to confirm correct gastric balloon positioning.

m. Add an additional 150 ml of air to the gastric balloon and reapply the clamp.

n. Irrigate the gastric port with saline. If no further gastric bleeding is found, leave the esophageal balloon deflated.

o. If bleeding persists, connect the esophageal balloon port to the pressure manometer and inflate the esophageal balloon to 25–45 mm Hg.

p. Transiently deflate the esophageal balloon every 4 hours to check for further bleeding (by aspirating through the gastric port) and to prevent ischemic necrosis of the esophageal mucosa.

q. Apply low intermittent suction to both the gastric and esophageal aspiration tubes.

r. After 24 hours without evidence of bleeding, deflate the esophageal and gastric balloons.

s. The SB tube can be removed after an additional 24 hours without evidence of bleeding.

7. Complications and Management:
    a. Esophageal perforation
        • Can result from intraesophageal inflation of the gastric balloon.
        • Deflate the gastric balloon and remove the SB tube.
        • Emergent surgical consult for operative therapy.
    b. Aspiration
        • Prevented by endotracheal intubation
        • Supportive therapy (oxygen, pulmonary toilet)
        • Antibiotics as indicated

c. Rebleeding
  - Reinsert SB tube
  - Transjugular intrahepatic portosystemic shunt, endoscopy, or definitive surgery

F. FEEDING TUBE TROUBLESHOOTING

Feeding tubes in either the stomach or the jejunum are frequently used in patients who cannot eat. They can be placed through open techniques, laparoscopically and endoscopically, but when they malfunction, a surgeon is usually called. It is critical that after manipulation of a feeding tube, its position within the lumen of the gut be verified either by aspiration of intestinal contents or by a contrast study through the tube. Failure to do so can cause tube feeds to be injected directly into the peritoneal cavity, which is life threatening.

1. Obstruction of Lumen

a. Prevented by flushing of tube with water or saline at regular intervals.
b. Avoid giving medications that are not easily liquefied through a feeding tube.
c. Clearing of obstruction should be attempted with saline or carbonated liquids using a 1-ml (tuberculin-type) syringe. A difficult clog can sometimes be broken up by injecting a carbonated beverage and capping the tube, and repeating this multiple times over the course of a day.
d. A guide wire can be used to break up inspissated tube feeds, but it must be used with extreme caution. It should be measured against the length of the feeding tube and not inserted more than 2–3 cm beyond the skin to prevent perforation of the bowel.
e. Crushed pancrease has been used to break up obstructing tube feeds.

2. Reinsertion of Feeding Tubes

a. Accidental removal is prevented by frequent inspection of the feeding tube to ensure that it is well secured.
b. Once a feeding tube has been in place for at least 2 weeks, if it falls out, reinsertion can usually be accomplished by passing a Foley catheter or MIC gastrostomy tube through the

previous wound and into the stomach or jejunum. This
should be done as soon as possible to prevent the tract from
closing.

  c. In the stomach, the balloon can be fully inflated. In the je-
     junum, the balloon should be inflated with no more than 2–3
     ml of saline to prevent intraluminal obstruction.
  d. A feeding tube that has been out for some time can often be
     replaced by interventional radiology. Insert a needle through
     the old site and place the feeding tube using the Seldinger
     technique under fluoroscopy.
  e. Placement must be confirmed radiographically.

3. Changing Feeding Tubes

  a. After approximately 1 month, the feeding tube tract is so
     well developed that the tube can be changed without fear of
     losing the tract.
  b. Feeding tubes can be changed simply by deflating the
     balloon, removing the tube, and replacing with a new
     tube.
  c. PEG tubes have a disc-like button in the stomach that can be
     difficult to extract through the skin wound. In these cases,
     the percutaneous endoscopic gastrostomy PEG tube should
     be changed or removed endoscopically.

4. Removing Feeding Tubes

  a. Feeding tubes should be left in place at least 2 weeks to en-
     sure that the bowel has "healed" to the abdominal wall so
     that there is no intra-abdominal leak after removing a feed-
     ing tube.
  b. The enterocutaneous fistula resulting from the feeding tube
     tract usually closes over time with conservative therapy.

II. LOWER GASTROINTESTINAL PROCEDURES

The anus and rectum are readily examined at the bedside
using a number of straightforward techniques. Likewise, many
lesions of the anorectal region are easily dealt with in the awake
patient without the need for general anesthesia or operating room
equipment. Although usually considered minor procedures, the
direct benefit to the patient is often immense.

A. ANOSCOPY

1. Indications:
  a. Anal lesions (fistulas, tumors, etc.)
  b. Rectal bleeding
  c. Rectal pain
  d. Banding or injection of hemorrhoids

2. Contraindications:
  a. Anal stricture
  b. Acute perirectal abscess
  c. Acutely thrombosed hemorrhoid

3. Anesthesia:
  None

4. Equipment:
  a. Clear polyethylene anoscope
  b. Water-soluble lubricant
  c. Directed light source or head-light

5. Positioning:
  Lateral decubitus position or lithotomy position

6. Technique:
  a. Examine anus by gently spreading anoderm and performing digital rectal examination.
  b. Insert the anoscope slowly, using a liberal amount of lubricant and with the obturator in place, until the flange at the base rests on perianal skin.
  c. Remove the obturator, and while withdrawing the anoscope, examine the anal mucosa in a systematic manner.
  d. Repeat the procedure as needed to ensure full inspection of the anal canal.

7. Complications and Management:
  a. Fissure
  • Anal or perianal tears may occur and usually respond to conservative measures.

b. Bleeding
  • Unusual, but may occur especially in the setting of large internal hemorrhoids; usually self-limited.

B. RIGID SIGMOIDOSCOPY

1. Indications:
  a. Rectal bleeding
  b. Lower abdominal and pelvic trauma
  c. Extraction of foreign bodies
  d. Stool cultures
  e. Evaluation and biopsy of ileoanal pouch

2. Contraindications:
  a. Anal stricture
  b. Acute perirectal abscess
  c. Acutely thrombosed hemorrhoids

3. Anesthesia:
  None

4. Equipment:
  a. Rigid sigmoidoscope and obturator
  b. Light source
  c. Suction apparatus
  d. Insufflating bulb
  e. Water-soluble lubricant
  f. Long cotton-tipped swabs
  g. Biopsy forceps, if desired

5. Positioning:
  Lateral decubitus, lithotomy, or prone jackknife

6. Technique:
  a. Administer tap water or saline enema before procedure to empty distal colon of feces.
  b. Perform a digital rectal examination to assess for masses.
  c. Assemble sigmoidoscope by placing the obturator through

the scope. Check light source and suction. Lubricate the scope thoroughly with water-soluble lubricant.

d. Gently insert the sigmoidoscope through the anus to 5 cm, remove the obturator, and attach the light source.

e. Judiciously insufflate air to visualize the lumen, using the minimum amount of air necessary to see.

f. Slowly advance the sigmoidoscope as a unit to visualize the rectum. Air will leak during the procedure, and intermittent insufflation will be necessary.

g. The lumen of the sigmoid will be posterior toward the sacrum and then gently curving to the patient's left. To minimize the risk of perforation, advance the sigmoidoscope only when the lumen is clearly visualized.

h. If stool is obstructing the view, use the cotton-tipped swabs to clear the lumen.

i. Advance the sigmoidoscope under direct vision as far as tolerated by the patient (most rigid scopes are 20 cm long) (see Figure 5.4).

j. To biopsy a mass or polyp, advance the scope until part of the mass is within the barrel of the scope. Insert the biopsy for-

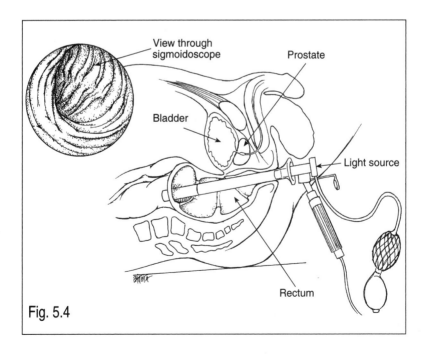

Fig. 5.4

ceps into the barrel, and grasp a specimen of tissue. If needed, silver nitrate sticks may be used to achieve hemostasis.

k. Systematically inspect the mucosa while withdrawing the instrument slowly.

7. Complications and Management:

a. Bleeding
- Usually self-limited, but may occur after biopsy.
- Rarely will require treatment, but if bleeding is hemodynamically significant, then resuscitate and consider endoscopic treatment.

b. Perforation
- Manifested by abdominal pain, distention, and loss of hepatic dullness to percussion.
- Obtain upright chest radiograph; free air under the diaphragm confirms the diagnosis.
- IV fluids, IV antibiotics, urgent operative management.

C. EXCISION OF THROMBOSED EXTERNAL HEMORRHOID

1. Indications:

Painful thrombosed external hemorrhoid

2. Contraindications:

a. Coagulopathy (PT or PTT >1.3× control)
b. Thrombocytopenia (platelet count < 50,000/mm^3)
c. Nonthrombosed prolapsed hemorrhoid

3. Anesthesia:

1% lidocaine (mixing lidocaine with 1/100,000 epinephrine may reduce bleeding)

4. Equipment:

a. Scalpel handle and #15 blade
b. Sterile prep solution
c. 25-gauge needle and syringe
d. Forceps
e. Small clamps
f. Vaseline or Xeroform gauze

5. Positioning:

Lateral decubitus or lithotomy

6. Technique:

a. Prep and drape the anal area with sterile prep solution.

b. Identify the thrombosed external hemorrhoid. By definition, it lies exterior to the dentate line, and it is firm and tender (see Figure 5.5).

c. Perform a field block of the hemorrhoid by infiltrating the surrounding skin and soft tissues with lidocaine using a 25-gauge needle.

d. Using a scalpel, make an elliptical incision over the thrombosed hemorrhoid (see Figure 5.6).

e. Using the forceps to hold one side of the incision, enucleate the clot within the hemorrhoid with the aid of a clamp. Apply a Vaseline gauze or Xeroform dressing.

f. The patient should be instructed to do sitz baths three times a day and after each bowel movement.

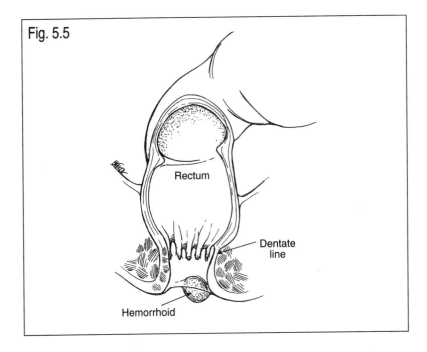

Fig. 5.5

Rectum

Dentate line

Hemorrhoid

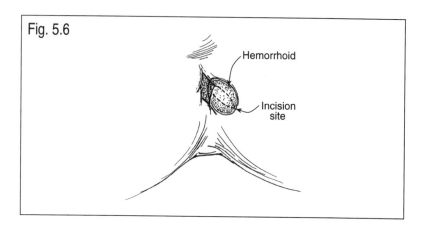

Fig. 5.6

7. Complications and Management:
   a. Bleeding
      • A small amount of dark bloody ooze is to be expected. Bright red bleeding indicates that the hemorrhoid is not thrombosed, and the incision should be stopped.
      • Direct pressure or packing may be required to control bleeding.
   b. Fissure
      • Usually results from extending the incision beyond the hemorrhoid into anoderm.
      • Treat conservatively with sitz baths and Anusol suppositories.
      • Manage operatively if conservative treatment fails.

D. REDUCTION OF RECTAL PROLAPSE

1. Indications:
   a. Prolapse of rectum (full-thickness)
   b. Mucosal prolapse of rectum (mucosa only)

2. Contraindications:
   a. Infarction or gangrene of prolapsed segment
   b. Severe tenderness of prolapsed segment
   c. Extreme edema of prolapsed segment

3. Anesthesia:
   None

4. Equipment:
   a. Gloves
   b. Water-soluble lubricant

5. Positioning:
   Decubitus or dorsal lithotomy

6. Technique:
   a. Don gloves and apply a liberal amount of water-soluble lubricant to the prolapsed segment.
   b. The concept is to apply steady, circumferential pressure on the prolapsed segment (to decrease edema) while simultaneously trying to reduce it. This is done by placing as many fingers of both hands as possible, oriented parallel to its longitudinal axis, around the segment and compressing it from all sides.
   c. Apply pressure firmly and steadily, with more pressure applied at the tip than at the base.
   d. Progress is typically slow and almost imperceptible. Be patient and squeeze for one to several minutes at a time, using plenty of lubricant.
   e. To prevent recurrence, the patient should be placed on stool softeners and should be instructed in the technique of manual self-reduction of prolapsed hemorrhoids, which may occur at each bowel movement.

7. Complications and Management:
   Unsuccessful reduction
   • May result in infarction of prolapsed segment
   • Requires surgical management with excision of prolapsed portion

III. ABDOMINAL PROCEDURES

These procedures are used to access the peritoneal cavity or to sample its contents. They are useful techniques that can provide diagnostic information or therapeutic benefit without the need for a major operative procedure.

A. PARACENTESIS

1. Indications:
   a. Diagnostic studies
   b. Ascites
   c. Spontaneous bacterial peritonitis
   d. Therapeutic purposes
   e. Relief of respiratory compromise
   f. Relief of abdominal pain and discomfort

2. Contraindications:
   a. Coagulopathy (PT or PTT > 1.3)
   b. Thrombocytopenia (plt < 60,000)
   c. Bowel obstruction
   d. Pregnancy
   e. Infected skin or soft tissue at entry site

3. Anesthesia:
   1% lidocaine

4. Equipment:
   a. Sterile prep solution
   b. Sterile towels
   c. Sterile gloves
   d. 5-ml syringes, 20-ml syringes, 25-gauge and 22-gauge needles
   e. 3-way stopcock, IV tubing
   f. IV catheter (diagnostic: 20-gauge, therapeutic: 18-gauge) or long 16-gauge (CVP-type) catheter with 0.035-cm J wire
   g. 500- to 1000-ml vacuum bottles and IV drip set (for therapeutic paracentesis)

5. Positioning:
   Supine
   a. Preferred sites of entry to prevent bleeding from epigastric vessels (see Figure 5.7)
      • Either lower quadrant (anterior iliac spine)
      • Lateral to the rectus muscle and at the level of or just below the umbilicus
      • Infraumbilically in the midline

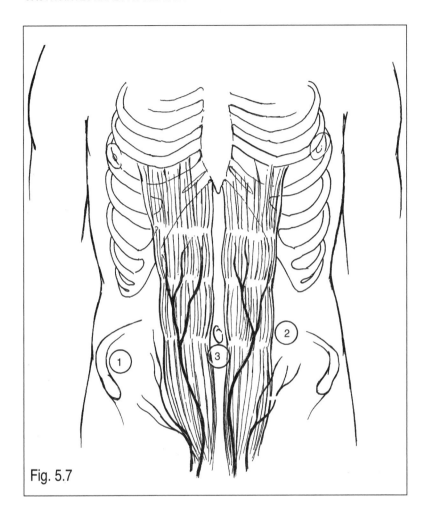

Fig. 5.7

b. The entry site should not be the site of a prior incision and should be free of gross contamination and infection.
c. The entry sites are percussed to confirm the presence of fluid and the absence of underlying bowel.
d. The patient should empty his or her bladder prior to the procedure, and/or a Foley catheter should be placed to decrease the possibility of puncturing the bladder.

6. Technique—Diagnostic Sampling:
   a. Prepare site with sterile prep solution and drape with sterile towels.

   b. Use 25-gauge needle to anesthetize skin and 22-gauge needle to anesthetize abdominal wall to peritoneum.

   c. Introduce IV catheter into the abdominal cavity, aspirating as it is advanced. The needle should traverse the abdominal wall at an oblique angle to prevent persistent leak of ascites from the puncture site (see Figure 5.8).

   d. When free flow of fluid occurs, the catheter should be advanced over the needle and the needle removed.

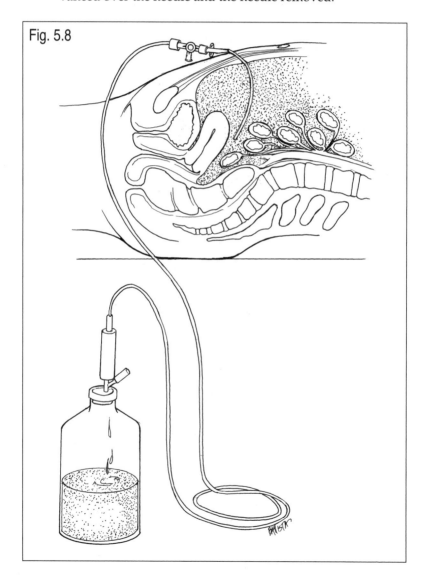

Fig. 5.8

e. Draw 20–30 ml of fluid into a sterile syringe for diagnostic studies and culture.

7. Technique—Therapeutic Drainage:

a. Prepare site with sterile prep solution and drape with sterile towels.

b. Use 25-gauge needle to anesthetize skin and 22-gauge needle to anesthetize abdominal wall to peritoneum.

c. Introduce IV catheter into the abdominal cavity, aspirating as it is advanced. The needle should traverse the abdominal wall at an oblique angle to prevent persistent leak of ascites from the puncture site.

d. When free flow of fluid occurs, the catheter should be advanced over the needle and the needle removed. Alternatively, a CVP-type catheter with extra side holes may be placed over a guide wire using the Seldinger technique.

e. After insertion of the needle and aspiration of fluid, a J-tip guide wire is placed through the needle into the peritoneal space. The needle is removed, leaving the wire in place.

f. A stiff plastic dilator is used to dilate the tract by placing it over the wire and into the abdomen. A #11-blade scalpel can be used to make a tiny nick at the entry site as well.

g. The dilator is removed, the catheter is placed over the wire and into the abdomen, and the wire is removed.

h. Draw 20–30 ml of fluid into a sterile syringe for diagnostic studies and culture.

i. IV tubing is hooked to the catheter and to a vacuum bottle to remove a large volume of fluid.

j. Should the catheter become occluded, careful manipulation of the catheter to re-establish flow may be undertaken. Alternatively, asking the patient to turn on his or her side and again onto his or her back may also help re-establish flow. However, the needle or guide wire should not be reintroduced because of the risk of bowel injury. If less than an adequate volume is withdrawn, the catheter should be removed and replaced, possibly at another entry site.

8. Complications and Management:

a. Hypotension
   • Can occur during or after procedure due to rapid mobilization of fluid from intravascular space or due to vasovagal response.

- IV hydration can prevent and correct the hypotension in most cases.
- 5% albumin solution or other colloid-based fluid is often used for this purpose.
  b. Bowel perforation
  - Rarely recognized at time of procedure
  - Can lead to infected ascites, peritonitis, and sepsis
  c. Hemorrhage
  - Rare, but can be caused by injury to mesentery or injury to inferior epigastric vessels.
  - Usually self-limited. Avoided by entering abdomen lateral to rectus and by correcting coagulopathy.
  - Hemodynamic instability requires laparotomy.
  d. Persistent ascites leak
  - Usually will seal in <2 weeks. Can result in peritonitis.
  - Skin entry site may be sutured to minimize leak.
  e. Bladder perforation
  - Avoided by inserting Foley catheter prior to procedure.
  - May require a period of bladder catheterization until sealed.
  - Obtain urology consult.

B. DIAGNOSTIC PERITONEAL LAVAGE

1. Indications:

Blunt abdominal trauma, in the setting of an equivocal or unreliable abdominal examination (e.g., after head trauma or intoxication) in a patient with unexplained hypotension or blood loss. It is particularly useful in a patient who is too unstable to transport for computed tomography (CT) scan or when CT is not available.

2. Absolute Contraindications:

a. Indication for laparotomy is already present
b. Pregnancy

3. Relative Contraindications:

a. Cirrhosis—Ascites can make the lavage fluid laboratory studies difficult to interpret.
b. Morbid obesity—Makes diagnostic peritoneal lavage (DPL) technically more difficult.

c. Prior abdominal surgery—Increases the risk of bowel injury during the procedure.

d. Suspected retroperitoneal injury—DPL results are often false-negative.

3. Anesthesia:

1% lidocaine with 1/100,000 epinephrine to decrease bleeding and false-positive results

4. Equipment:

a. Sterile prep solution
b. Sterile towels, sterile gloves, gown, mask, cap
c. Syringes: 5 ml, 10 ml, 20 ml
d. 25-gauge needle
e. Peritoneal dialysis catheter
f. IV tubing
g. 1000-ml bag of normal saline or Ringer's lactate
h. Scalpel handle and #10 and #11 (or #15) blades
i. Surgical instruments: tissue forceps, hemostats, Allis clamps, retractors, suture

5. Positioning:

Supine. The stomach should be decompressed by an NG or an OG tube (OG if head trauma is present). The bladder should be drained by a Foley catheter.

6. Technique:

a. Prepare the entire abdomen with sterile prep solution and drape with sterile towels.
b. With a 25-gauge needle and lidocaine with epinephrine, anesthetize a site in the lower midline approximately one-third the distance from the umbilicus to the symphysis pubis (see Figure 5.9).
c. Make a small incision down to the linea alba (the linea alba is midline in position and recognized by its decussating fibers and absence of muscle beneath it).
d. Incise the fascia and peritoneum in the midline for a length of approximately 1 cm, grasping the edges of the fascia with hemostats or Allis clamps (see Figure 5.10).
e. Introduce the dialysis catheter into the peritoneal cavity at

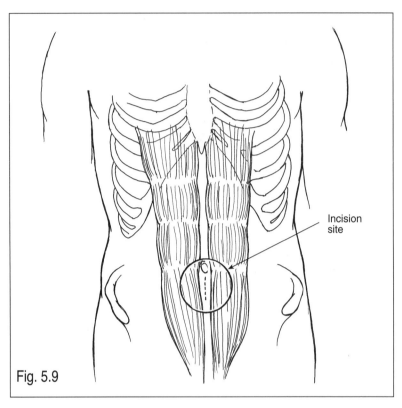

Incision
site

Fig. 5.9

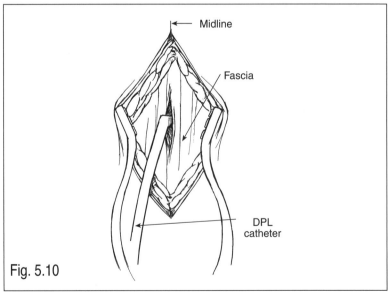

Midline

Fascia

DPL
catheter

Fig. 5.10

an oblique angle aiming toward the cul-de-sac, and advance it carefully into the pelvis.

f. Aspirate from the catheter with a syringe. Gross blood (5 ml or more) or gross enteric contents are indications for immediate laparotomy.

g. If no gross blood or enteric contents are aspirated, instill 10 ml/kg of warmed saline or Ringer's lactate, up to 1000 ml, via the IV tubing. Drainage of dialysate into a chest tube or Foley catheter is also an indication for laparotomy.

h. After waiting 5–10 minutes, allow the fluid to drain by gravity back into its original bag.

i. Send a sample of the fluid for cell count and amylase. Positive findings include a red blood cell count of >100,000/mm^3, a white blood cell count >500/mm^3, or amylase >175.

j. Note: Criteria for positive lavage findings may vary among individual trauma surgeons.

k. At the conclusion of the procedure, the catheter is removed and the fascia and skin are closed carefully using standard techniques (interrupted #1 Prolene, Vicryl, or PDS suture for fascia).

7. Complications and Management:

a. Bladder injury
- Preventable by inserting Foley catheter prior to procedure.
- Treated by Foley catheter drainage for a period of several days.

b. Injury to bowel or other abdominal organ
- Treated with nothing-by-mouth status, IV hydration, and IV antibiotics.
- Bowel perforation with soilage requires laparotomy for repair.

c. Hemorrhage
- Rarely life-threatening, but may lead to false-positive results, especially if source is skin or subcutaneous tissue.
- Treated with nothing-by-mouth status, IV hydration, transfusion, and laparotomy if it persists.

d. Peritonitis
- May be due to poor aseptic technique or bowel perforation.
- Laparotomy may be necessary to rule out perforation.

e. Wound infection
- A potential late complication. Incidence may be

diminished by a dose of broad-spectrum IV antibiotics prior to procedure.
• Treated with antibiotics and by opening the wound and packing it.

C. TENCKHOFF CATHETER INSERTION

1. Indications:

Short-term or chronic ambulatory peritoneal dialysis

2. Contraindications:

a. Obliterated peritoneal space (prior surgery, infection, carcinomatosis)
b. Ruptured diaphragm
c. Respiratory insufficiency
d. Presence of a large ventral or umbilical hernia

3. Anesthesia:

1% lidocaine (1/100,000 epinephrine may reduce bleeding)

4. Equipment:

a. Surgical prep solution, sterile towels, sterile gloves
b. Scalpel handle and #10 blade
c. Tissue forceps
d. Self-retaining retractor
e. Double-cuff peritoneal dialysis catheter
f. 3–0 absorbable suture on a taper-point curved needle
g. 2–0 nylon suture on a curved cutting needle
h. 25-gauge and 22-gauge needle
i. 10-ml syringe

5. Positioning:

Supine. The stomach should be decompressed by an NG or an OG tube. The bladder should be drained by a Foley catheter.

6. Technique:

a. Prepare the entire abdomen with sterile prep solution and drape with sterile towels.
b. With a 25-gauge needle and lidocaine, anesthetize a site lat-

eral to the midline (over the rectus abdominus) approximately one-third the distance from the umbilicus to the symphysis pubis.

c. Make a longitudinal incision approximately 5 cm in length down to the level of fascia.

d. Anesthetize a tract for the creation of a subcutaneous tunnel, to a point 8–12 cm lateral to the incision, and make a small stab incision at this point (see Figure 5.11).

e. Tunnel the dialysis catheter such that the proximal cuff lies in a subcutaneous location and the distal cuff lies in the first incision (see Figure 5.12).

f. Make an incision in the fascia and retract the rectus laterally, exposing the posterior fascia.

g. Place a purse-string of 3–0 absorbable suture in the posterior fascia (see Figure 5.13).

h. Under direct vision, carefully incise the posterior fascia and peritoneum in the center of the purse-string suture. Locally

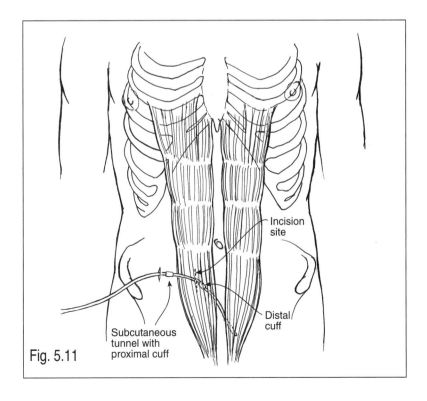

Fig. 5.11

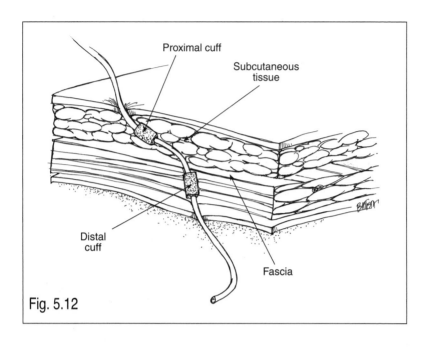

Fig. 5.12

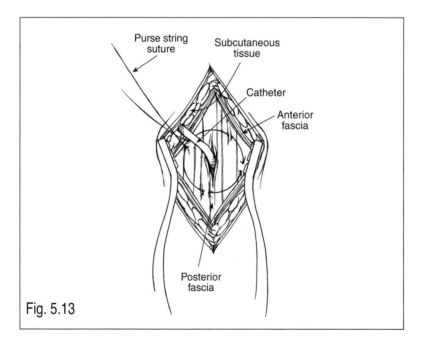

Fig. 5.13

Fig. 5.14

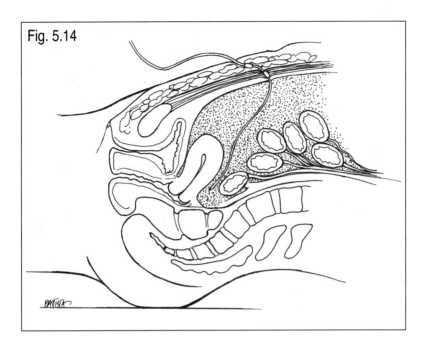

explore the peritoneal cavity to be certain that adhesions or viscera are not in the way.

i. Carefully insert the catheter into the peritoneal cavity, aiming inferiorly and posteriorly, such that the distal cuff lies just anterior to the peritoneum. The catheter should feed easily and without resistance into the pelvis. Flush the catheter with heparinized saline (100 units/ml) and be certain of the lack of significant resistance (see Figure 5.14).

j. Secure the catheter with the purse-string suture.

k. Close the anterior fascia around the catheter such that the cuff lies within the muscle.

l. The skin may be closed in the usual fashion.

m. Secure the catheter where it exits the smaller incision with skin sutures.

n. The function of the catheter should be tested by infusing 1 l of saline or Ringer's lactate and then allowing it to drain by gravity.

o. Peritoneal dialysis can begin the same day, using small volumes (1 L).

7. Complications and Management:

   a. Injury to intra-abdominal viscus
      - May occur in the setting of extensive adhesions or previous surgery
   b. Peritonitis
      - An ever-present risk that requires careful technique and surveillance
      - Treated with IV and/or intraperitoneal antibiotics
      - May occasionally require removal of catheter
   c. Catheter dysfunction
      - May be caused by ingrowth of tissue or adhesions to the catheter, and usually requires catheter removal.
      - If it is placed correctly deep in the pelvis, catheter is less likely to be occluded by omentum.

CHAPTER **6**

NEUROSURGICAL PROCEDURES

Author: Kevin A. Walter, M.D.

NEUROSURGICAL PROCEDURES

A. LUMBAR PUNCTURE

1. Indications:
    a. Cerebrospinal fluid (CSF) evaluation
        • Meningitis
        • Subarachnoid hemorrhage
        • Neoplastic disease
    b. CSF drainage
        • Communicating hydrocephalus
        • Pseudotumor cerebri
        • CSF leak
    c. Intracranial pressure measurement
        • Communicating hydrocephalus
        • Pseudotumor cerebri
    d. Intrathecal drug administration
        • Radiopaque contrast
        • Antibiotics
        • Antineoplastic chemotherapy

2. Contraindications:
    All patients should receive intracranial imaging (computed tomography [CT] or magnetic resonance [MR]) to rule out an intracranial mass lesion prior to lumbar puncture.
    a. Noncommunicating hydrocephalus
    b. Intracranial mass (tumor, abscess, hematoma)
    c. Coagulopathy or platelets <50K

    d. Cellulitis at intended puncture site
    e. Complete spinal block above tap site
    f. Tethered cord syndrome

3. Anesthesia:

    Lidocaine (0.5%, 1.0%, or 2.0%)

4. Equipment:

    a. Sterile prep solution
    b. Sterile gloves and towels
    c. 22-gauge and 25-gauge needles
    d. 22-gauge, 20-gauge, or 18-gauge spinal needle with stylet
    e. CSF collection vials
    f. Manometer with stopcock

5. Positioning:

    a. Lateral: Patient is placed on his or her side with chin and
       knees tucked into the chest. This position is favored for accu-
       rate measurement of intracranial pressure (fetal position—
       see Figure 6.1).
    b. Sitting: Patient sits on the side of a bed, flexed forward over
       a pillow for support. Intracranial pressure cannot be mea-
       sured in this position. This position is superior for obese pa-
       tients (see Figure 6.2).

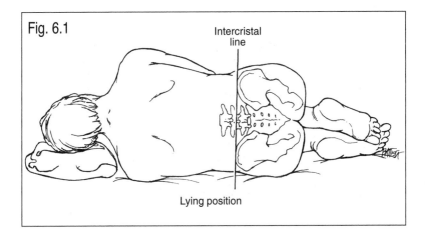

Fig. 6.1

Intercristal line

Lying position

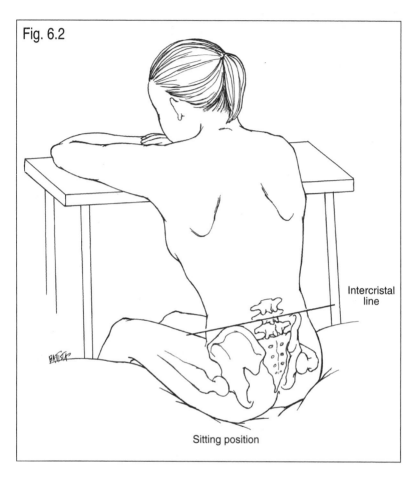

Fig. 6.2

Intercristal line

Sitting position

6. Technique:

   a. Apply sterile prep solution to the lower back and cover region with sterile drapes.

   b. Identify the target interspace. The L4-5 interspace falls in the midline along the intercristal line connecting the superior iliac crests. Lumbar puncture may be attempted at the L3-4, L4-5, and L5-S1 interspaces.

   c. Inject 1 ml of lidocaine subcutaneously into the target interspace to raise a skin wheal. Anesthetize the deep tissues by injecting 3 ml of lidocaine through the skin wheal with a 22-gauge needle. Follow the intended track of the lumbar puncture needle, directed slightly cranially and parallel to the midline.

   d. Insert the spinal needle along the anesthetized tract with the stylet in place. The bevel of the needle should face laterally (i.e., toward the ceiling in the lateral position) (see Figure 6.3).

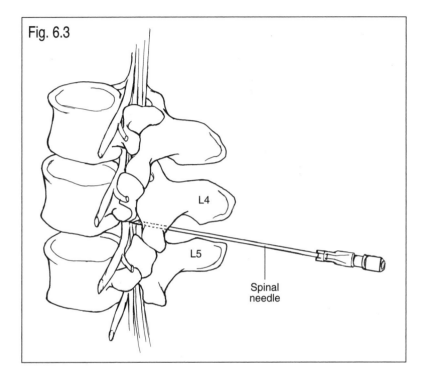

Fig. 6.3

L4

L5

Spinal needle

e. Advance the needle deeper, aiming rostrally about 15°, taking care to maintain a midline trajectory. The needle will encounter slight resistance, then a pop will be felt, representing penetration through the ligamentum flavum (yellow ligament) into the thecal sac (the stylet should always be used with needle to prevent introduction of epidermal cells or subcutaneous tissue into thecal sac) (see Figure 6.4).

f. If bone is encountered, pull the needle back to the subcutaneous tissues. The tip of the needle must be above the dorsal lumbar fascia to successfully redirect. Confirm that the trajectory is in the midline and that the patient is adequately flexed to open the interspace. If bone is encountered a second time, use the needle to "march" cranially to caudally until the thecal sac is entered. If this technique is unsuccessful, try another interspace or reposition the patient for the sitting approach.

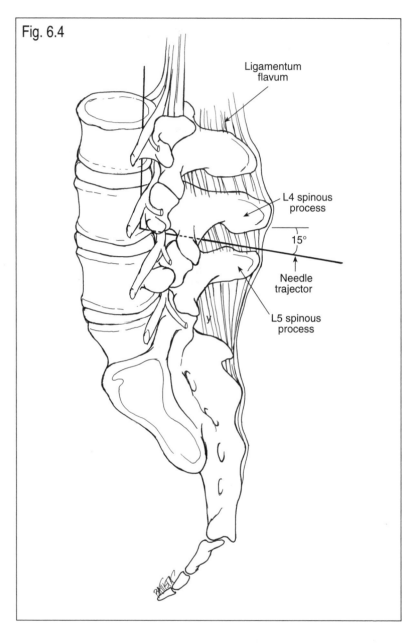

Fig. 6.4

Ligamentum flavum

L4 spinous process

15°

Needle trajector

L5 spinous process

g. Once the needle is in the thecal sac, remove the stylet and observe for CSF (see Figure 6.5). If blood appears, allow blood to drain and observe for clearance. If blood clears, then the tap was traumatic. If blood does not clear and blood clots, re-

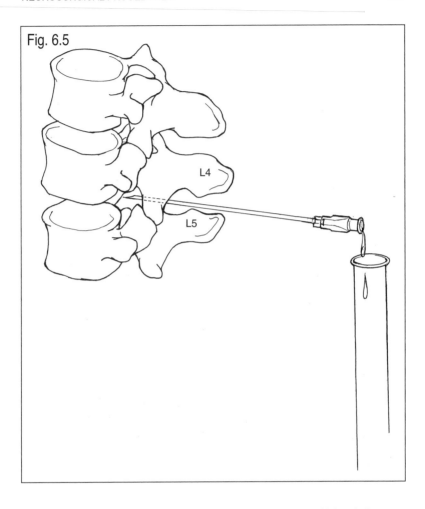

Fig. 6.5

place stylet, withdraw needle, and reattempt. If blood does not clear and does not clot, the patient may have had a subarachnoid hemorrhage and samples should be sent to the laboratory for cell counts and examined for xanthochromia.

h. Once CSF flow is established, place stopcock on end of spinal needle with manometer. Rotate spinal needle so that bevel is pointed cranially. Open stopcock and measure CSF pressure in cm H2O (Normal <15 cm H_2O; borderline 15–20 cm H_2O; abnormal >20 cm H_2O).

i. Collect CSF samples in tubes. The following tubes should be sent for analysis on every lumbar puncture performed:
   • Cell count
   • Protein and glucose

- Culture and sensitivity
- Cell count (to compare with first cell count)

j. Replace stylet and withdraw needle.
k. Place sterile gauze over puncture site. Changes in mental status, vital signs, and pupil size and reactivity must be carefully monitored.

7. Complications and Management:

a. Tonsillar herniation
- Manifests initially as altered mental status, followed by cranial nerve abnormalities (third nerve palsy, respiratory difficulties) and Cushing response (hypertension, bradycardia, respiratory depression). May be rapidly fatal.
- Immediately remove needle and raise the head of bed to improve venous return from the brain.
- Administer 1 g/kg of mannitol intravenously.
- Intubate patient and hyperventilate to a goal $PCO_2 = 30$ mm Hg.
- Emergent neurosurgical consult.

b. Nerve root injury
- Withdraw needle immediately.
- If pain or motor weakness persists, start corticosteroids (Decadron 4 mg every 6 hours).
- Electromyogram/nerve conduction velocity studies should be scheduled if pain persists.

c. Spinal headache
- Keep the patient supine as tolerated.
- Usually resolves within hours but can persist for days.
- Hydration and caffeine may help ameliorate symptoms.

d. Aortic/arterial puncture
- Withdraw needle immediately and keep the patient supine for 4–6 hours while monitoring hemodynamics.
- Vascular surgery consult.

B. LUMBAR DRAIN PLACEMENT

1. Indications:

a. CSF fistula or CSF leak
b. Intrathecal pressure monitoring
- Pseudotumor cerebri
- Normal pressure hydrocephalus
- Aortic surgery

     c. Communicating hydrocephalus
- Subarachnoid hemorrhage
- Meningitis

2. Contraindications:

All patients should receive intracranial imaging (CT or MR) to rule out an intracranial mass lesion prior to lumbar puncture.
  a. Noncommunicating hydrocephalus
  b. Intracranial mass (tumor, abscess, hematoma)
  c. Coagulopathy or platelets <50K
  d. Infection in the region of puncture
  e. Complete spinal block above lesion
  f. Tethered cord syndrome

3. Anesthesia:

lidocaine (0.5%, 1.0%, 2.0%)

4. Equipment:

  a. Sterile prep solution
  b. Sterile gloves and towels
  c. 14-gauge Touhy needle
  d. IV pressure tubing
  e. Lumbar drain
  f. CSF collection bag (e.g., bile bag)
  g. Ruler

5. Positioning:

The patient must be in the lateral position with the knees and chin tucked into the chest (fetal position—see Figure 6.6).

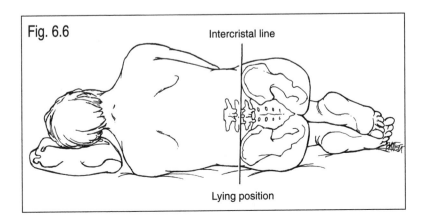

Fig. 6.6

Intercristal line

Lying position

6. Technique:

a. Apply sterile prep solution to the lower back and cover region with sterile drapes.

b. Identify the target interspace. The L4-5 interspace falls in the midline along the intercristal line connecting the superior iliac crests. Lumbar puncture may be attempted at the L3-4, L4-5, and L5-S1 interspaces.

c. Inject 1 ml of lidocaine subcutaneously into the target interspace to raise a skin wheal. Anesthetize the deep tissues by injecting 3 ml of lidocaine through the skin wheal with a 22-gauge needle. Follow the intended track of the Touhy needle, directed slightly cranially and parallel to the midline.

d. Insert the Touhy needle along the anesthetized tract with the stylet in place. The bevel of the needle should face laterally (i.e., toward the ceiling in the lateral position).

e. Advance the needle in the midline while aiming 15° rostrally. The needle will encounter slight resistance, then a pop will be felt, representing penetration through the ligamentum flavum (yellow ligament) into the thecal sac (the stylet should always be used with needle to prevent introduction of epidermoid cells or subcutaneous tissue into thecal sac).

f. If bone is encountered, pull the needle back to the subcutaneous tissues. The tip of the needle must be above the dorsal lumbar fascia to successfully redirect. Confirm that the trajectory is in the midline and that the patient is adequately flexed to open the interspace. If bone is encountered a second time, use the needle to "march" cranially to caudally until the thecal sac is entered. If this technique is unsuccessful, try another interspace.

g. Once the needle is in the thecal sac, remove the stylet and observe for CSF (see Figure 6.7). If blood appears, allow blood to drain and observe for clearance. If blood clears, then tap was traumatic. If blood does not clear and blood clots, replace stylet, withdraw needle, and reattempt.

h. If CSF flow is established, slowly withdraw stylet and feed 10 cm of the lumbar drain through the Touhy needle. The drain should now be in the thecal space (see Figure 6.8).

i. Slowly withdraw the Touhy needle over the lumbar drain, taking care to ensure the drain does not move.

j. CSF should be dripping from the lumbar drain.

k. Place the connector to the free end of the drain and connect to IV pressure tubing (see Figure 6.9).

l. Secure the drain to the patient's back with sterile dressing.

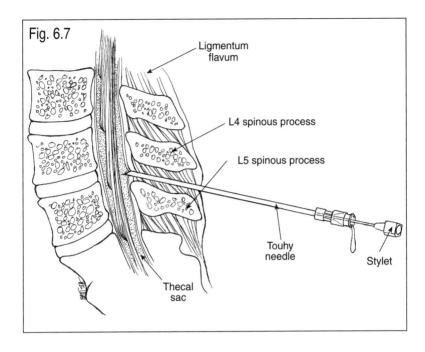

Fig. 6.7

Ligmentum flavum

L4 spinous process

L5 spinous process

Touhy needle

Stylet

Thecal sac

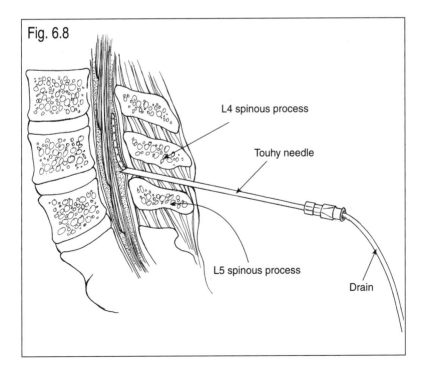

Fig. 6.8

L4 spinous process

Touhy needle

L5 spinous process

Drain

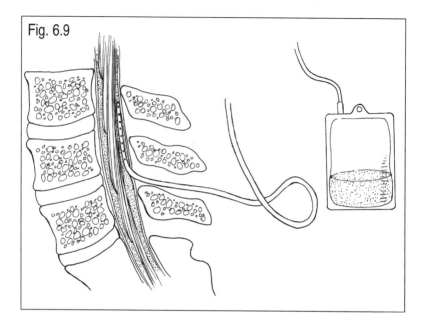

Fig. 6.9

m. Lay the patient supine and set the desired drainage pressure using a ruler. The collection bag is placed at a given height above the lower back (e.g., the standard is a "pop-off" of 10 cm. To achieve this, the bag should be placed 10 cm above the lower back).

n. The pop-off may be adjusted up or down to achieve a desired rate of CSF drainage. Generally no more than 15 ml of CSF should be drained per hour or a spectrum of symptoms beginning with headache and progressing through lethargy, coma, and death may ensue.

7. Complications and Management:

a. Tonsillar herniation
   - Manifests initially as altered mental status, followed by cranial nerve abnormalities (third nerve palsy) and Cushing response (hypertension, bradycardia, respiratory depression). May be rapidly fatal.
   - Immediately remove needle and raise the head of bed to improve venous return from the brain.
   - Administer 1 g/kg of mannitol intravenously.
   - Intubate patient and hyperventilate to a goal $P_{CO_2} = 30$ mm Hg.
   - Emergent neurosurgical consult.

   b. Nerve root injury
      • Withdraw needle immediately.
      • If pain or motor weakness persists, start corticosteroids
        (Decadron 4 mg every 6 hours).
      • Electromyogram/nerve conduction velocity studies should
        be scheduled if pain persists.
   c. Spinal headache
      • Keep the patient supine as tolerated.
      • Usually resolves within hours but can persist for days.
      • Hydration and caffeine may help ameliorate symptoms.
   d. Aortic/arterial puncture
      • Withdraw needle immediately and keep the patient supine
        for 4–6 hours while monitoring hemodynamics.
      • Vascular surgery consult.
   e. Meningitis
      • Obtain CSF cultures from the drain, and then remove the
        drain and culture the intrathecal portion.
      • Start broad-spectrum antibiotics, for example, vancomycin
        and a third-generation cephalosporin.

C. VENTRICULOSTOMY/INTRACRANIAL PRESSURE (ICP) MONITOR (BOLT) PLACEMENT

1. Indications:

   Placement of ventriculostomy/subarachnoid bolt as a bedside
procedure should be performed only in patients with the following
criteria:
   a. Clinical signs of impending brain stem herniation
   b. Cushing triad
   c. Third nerve palsy
   d. Radiographic signs of impending brain stem herniation
   e. Uncal herniation
   f. Tonsillar herniation
   g. Severe subfalcine herniation
   h. Severely impaired mental status (Glasgow Coma Score
      (GCS) < 8)
Because of the significant risk of infection and intracranial
hemorrhage associated with this procedure, patients who are not
critically ill, but who require ventriculostomy/bolt placement
should have this procedure performed in the operating room on an
urgent basis. Ventriculostomy/bolt placement is a bedside
procedure only in life-threatening situations.

2. Contraindications:

    a. Coagulopathy/thrombocytopenia
    b. Age <1 year (see ventricular tap following)
    Other relative contraindications exist for these procedures;
however, they do not apply in the life-threatening situations
outlined previously.

3. Anesthesia:

    1% lidocaine, short-acting IV sedation, and nondepolarizing
paralytics if patient is moving. If the patient is conscious enough to
prevent you from performing this procedure, it should not be
performed at the bedside.

4. Equipment:

    a. Sterile prep solution
    b. Sterile gloves and towels
    c. 22-gauge and 25-gauge needles
    d. 22-gauge spinal needle with stylet
    e. Two razors
    f. Bone wax
    g. Sterile saline solution
    h. Scalpel
    i. 3–0 nylon suture
    j. Needle driver
    k. Scissors
    l. Hand-held cranial twist drill
    m. Standard ventricular catheter or Richmond bolt and/or in-
       traparenchymal ICP monitoring device (e.g., Camino)
    n. Sterile dressing

5. Positioning:

    The patient should be supine with the head of the bed raised
20° to 25°. The head should be in the neutral position (see Figure
6.10).

6. Technique

    a. Shave the anterior one-fourth of the scalp on the side the
       drain/bolt is to be placed (from the midline laterally to the
       external acoustic meatus).
    b. Kocher's point is the most commonly used site for
       drain/bolt placement (see Figure 6.11). This lies anterior to

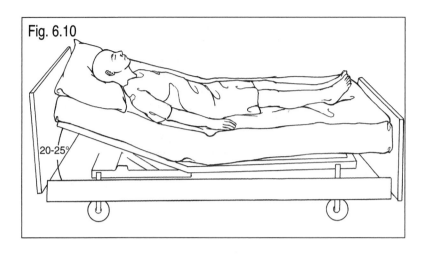

Fig. 6.10

20-25°

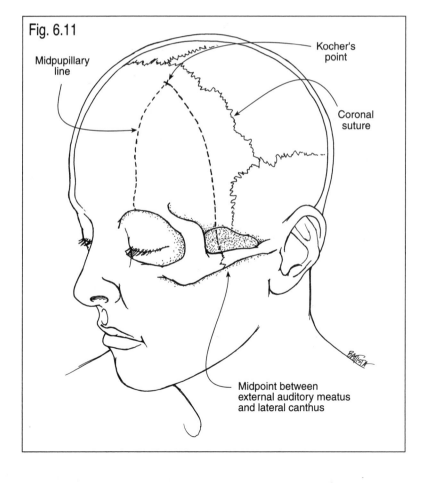

Fig. 6.11

Midpupillary line

Kocher's point

Coronal suture

Midpoint between external auditory meatus and lateral canthus

the motor homunculus and avoids injury to the superior sagittal sinus. To find Kocher's point, follow a perpendicular line up midway between the external auditory meatus and lateral canthus of the eye to intersect the midpupillary line. Alternatively, if the coronal suture is palpable, mark the intersection 2 cm anterior to the coronal suture and 4 cm lateral to midline. Although either the right or left Kocher's point may be used, typically the right is chosen because it represents the nondominant hemisphere. Indications for placement of a left Kocher's point ventriculostomy/bolt include focal lesion (tumor, trauma, arteriovenous malformation) in the pathway of the catheter inserted on the right or presence of significant intraventricular hemorrhage in the right lateral ventricle (which would likely clog the catheter).

c. Perform a 5-minute sterile prep of the shaved areas.

d. Drape the intended placement site, taking care to clearly define the midline.

e. Make a 2-cm parasagittal incision over Kocher's point down to bone using the scalpel to scrape away and elevate the pericranium.

f. Use the twist drill to carefully make a hole in the skull, taking care not to plunge into the brain (see Figure 6.12).

g. Irrigate away the bone chips with saline solution and use bone wax to stop bone bleeding.

h. Puncture the underlying dura with the spinal needle and widen the dural incision a few millimeters (see Figure 6.13).

i. Insert ventricular catheter (IVC) with stylet perpendicular to brain surface to depth of 5 to 7 cm. A palpable pop should be felt as the catheter enters the ventricle. Do not insert catheter more than 7 cm (see Figure 6.14).

j. Withdraw the stylet to ensure CSF flow. If no CSF flow is established, lower the distal end of the catheter because the pressure may be low. If still no CSF is obtained, gradually withdraw catheter from brain and watch for flow as the catheter is withdrawn. If no CSF is seen and the catheter is entirely withdrawn, pass the catheter again with stylet in place and redirect slightly toward the midline (see Figure 6.15).

k. If unsuccessful in obtaining CSF after three attempts, place a subarachnoid bolt or intraparenchymal monitor instead.

• For the Richmond bolt, screw in until the tip is flush with the inner table of the skull (see Figure 6.16).

• For the Camino or other intraparenchymal monitoring

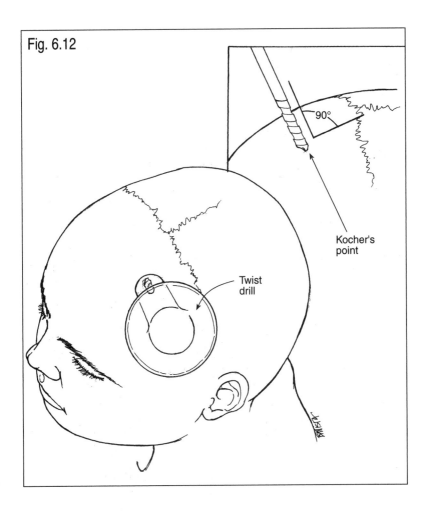

Fig. 6.12

90°

Kocher's point

Twist drill

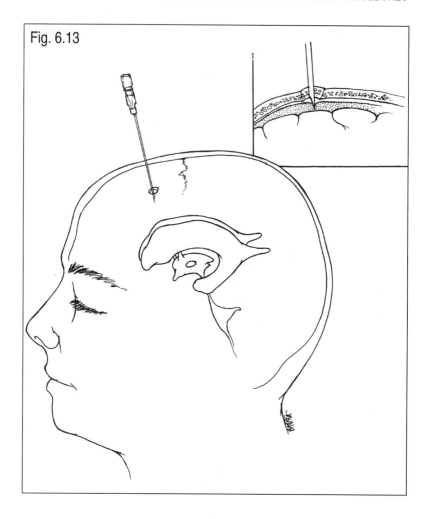

Fig. 6.13

device, screw in stabilizing bolt and insert device 1.5 to 2 cm through the burr hole into the brain parenchyma
- Note: The radius of the Richmond screw or Camino monitor must match the radius of the twist drill used to make the burr hole, otherwise the bolt will not form an adequate seal. Each monitoring device should screw easily into an appropriate size burr hole. The monitor should not be able to be removed from the burr hole without unscrewing the bolt.
1. Connect the IVC or ICP monitor to the pressure transducer and/or drainage level. Set a fixed pop-off level for drainage

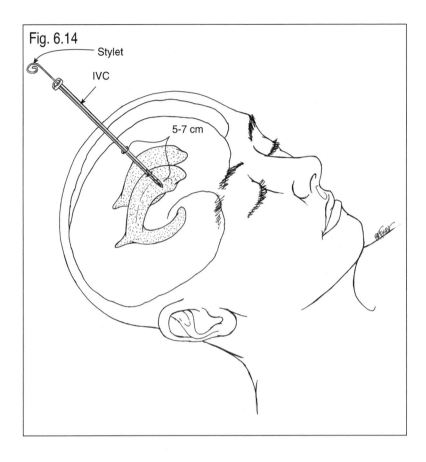

Fig. 6.14
Stylet
IVC
5-7 cm

using the ear as reference (place the bag 10 cm above the ear). (see Figure 6.9)

m. Suture all incisions and secure IVC drain to scalp.

n. Use sterile dressing over entire frontal portion of scalp.

7. Complications and Management:

a. Bleeding

- If there is any change in neurological examination, seizure, or unexpected blood seen after placement of IVC, an immediate head CT should be obtained.

- Most IVC hemorrhages resolve spontaneously and require supportive care. Occasionally, the CT may reveal an aberrantly placed IVC that needs removal.

- In very rare circumstances, operative evacuation of hematoma is indicated.

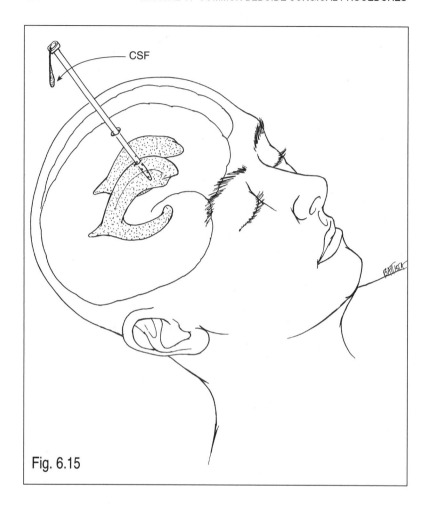

Fig. 6.15

b. Infection
- The reported risk of infection varies from 0 to 27%. CSF surveillance cultures should be taken if the patient is febrile and prior to drain removal.
- Antibiotic coverage for skin flora is given prophylactically (e.g., oxacillin). Aggressive antibiotics (vancomycin with a third-generation cephalosporin) are given in cases of presumed ventriculitis. Intraventricular aminoglycosides may be helpful for gram-negative infections.
- All IVCs and ICP monitors should be removed after 1 week and replaced if still needed to reduce infection risk.

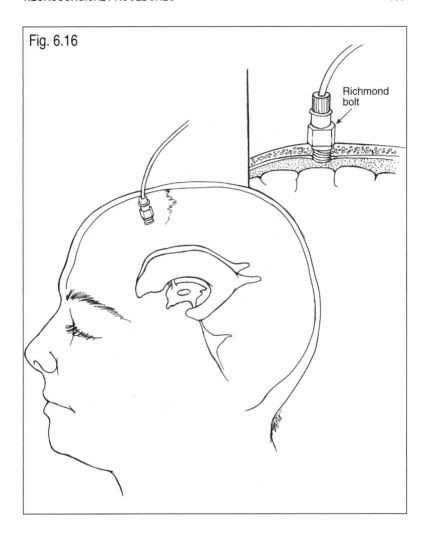

Fig. 6.16

c. Tonsillar herniation
   • Can manifest as dilating unilateral pupil, change in mental
     status, Cushing triad (hypertension, bradycardia, decrease
     respiratory rate).
   • Immediately clamp off IVC.
   • Intubate and hyperventilation.
   • Mannitol (0.5–1 g/kg) and other diuretics.
   • Emergent neurosurgery consult.
d. Aneurysm rupture
   • If bright red blood is suddenly seen draining from IVC,
     emergently place another IVC in the other ventricle to

maintain ventricular access.
- Set pop-off to 20 mm Hg to prevent herniation but minimize excessive drainage.
- Emergent head CT.
- Emergent neurosurgery consult.

D. EMERGENT PERCUTANEOUS VENTRICULAR PUNCTURE

1. Indications:
   a. Infant <1 year with open cranial sutures
   b. Life-threatening herniation from hydrocephalus
   c. Life-threatening ventriculoperitoneal (VP) shunt malfunction

2. Contraindications:

   Coagulopathy

3. Anesthesia:

   None

4. Equipment:
   a. Sterile prep solution
   b. Sterile gloves and towels
   c. 22-gauge spinal needles

5. Positioning:

   Supine

6. Technique:

   Palpate anterior fontanelle
   a. Shave hair and sterile prep over fontanelle.
   b. With the spinal needle, pierce the scalp and dura as far later-ally along the coronal suture as possible to prevent injury to superior sagittal sinus.
   c. Advance needle 2 to 3 cm into ventricle.
   d. Pull out stylet and observe for CSF. If no CSF, replace stylet and advance needle further 1 cm.
   e. If still no CSF, pull out the needle and reaim trajectory.

7. Complications and Management:
   a. Bleeding
      • If there is any change in neurological examination, seizure, or unexpected blood seen after placement of the catheter, an immediate head CT should be obtained.
      • Most hemorrhages resolve spontaneously and require supportive care.
      • In rare circumstances, operative evacuation of hematoma is indicated.
   b. Tonsillar herniation
      • Can manifest as dilating unilateral pupil, change in mental status, Cushing triad (hypertension, bradycardia, decrease respiratory rate).
      • Immediately remove the needle.
      • Intubate and hyperventilation.
      • Mannitol (0.5–1 g/kg) and other diuretics.
      • Emergent neurosurgery consult.

E. SHUNT TAP

Ventriculoperitoneal (VP), ventriculoatrial (VA) and ventriculopleural shunts are commonly encountered neurosurgical devices used for chronic CSF diversion. A shunt tap is often required to evaluate for shunt problems.

1. Indications:
   a. Obtain CSF for analysis
   b. Evaluate shunt function
   c. Measure intraventricular pressure
   d. Temporizing measure to remove CSF in a distally occluded shunt
   e. Injection of antibiotic or chemotherapeutic agents
   f. Injection of contrast agents

2. Contraindications:
   a. Scalp infection around shunt site
   b. Severe coagulopathy or platelets <25K
   c. Collapsed or slit ventricles

3. Anesthesia:
   None usually needed

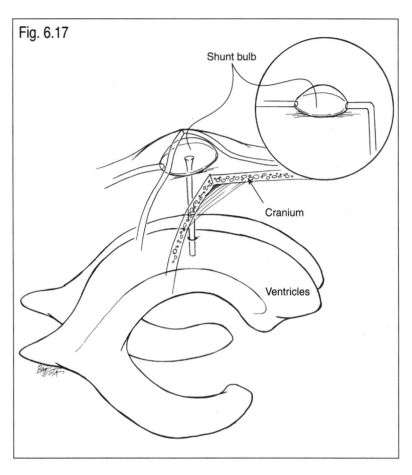

Fig. 6.17

Shunt bulb

Cranium

Ventricles

4. Equipment:
    a. Sterile prep solution
    b. Sterile gloves and towels
    c. 25-gauge or 23-gauge butterfly needles
    d. 10-ml syringe
    e. Manometer with stopcock

5. Positioning:
    Supine

6. Technique:
    a. Palpate scalp for shunt bulb, which is usually in the right frontal or right occipital regions within 2 cm of the scalp inci-

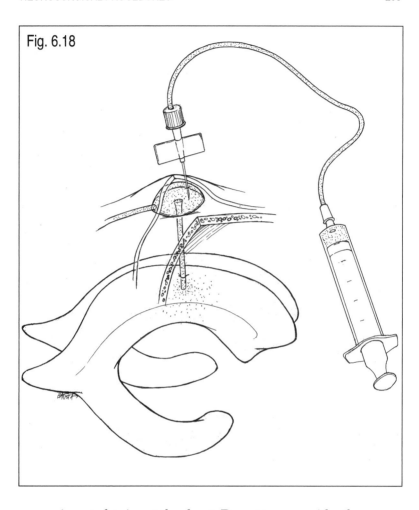

Fig. 6.18

sion used to insert the shunt. Do not tamper with other shunt components because this may affect shunt function (Figure 6.17).

b. Shave and prep the area for 5 minutes.

c. Introduce the butterfly needle into bulb at a slight oblique angle and observe for spontaneous flow of CSF into tubing (Figure 6.18).

d. Attach stopcock with manometer to end of tubing, ensuring that the zero level on the manometer is level with the bulb. Alternately, if no manometer is available, the distance that CSF travels up the butterfly tubing when held vertically may be measured.

e. If no spontaneous CSF flow is observed, take 5-ml syringe and

gently attempt to aspirate CSF. If CSF is aspirated easily, then the ventricular pressure is at or near zero. If CSF is difficult to aspirate or no CSF is obtained, then the proximal end of the shunt is occluded or the ventricles are collapsed, and aborting the procedure is necessary.
f. Send CSF for laboratory analysis.
g. Inject chemotherapeutic or antimicrobial agent if desired.
h. Withdraw needle and hold gentle pressure over bulb.

7. Complications and Management:
a. Ventriculitis
  • Every time the shunt is manipulated, there is a chance of introducing infection into the system.
  • In patients with systemic infection with no obvious central nervous system source whose shunt was placed more than 2 months prior to the date of the intended tap, a lumbar puncture should be performed rather than a shunt tap to reduce the chance of seeding the shunt.
b. Occlusion
  • In patients with collapsed or slit-like ventricles, attempting to aspirate CSF can cause occlusion of the proximal shunt. A head CT should always be obtained prior to shunt tap to minimize the risk of this complication.

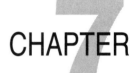

CHAPTER 7

UROLOGIC PROCEDURES

Author: Misop Han, M.D.

UROLOGIC PROCEDURES

I. UROLOGY

The specialty of urology involves the evaluation and treatment of various disorders and diseases of the male genitourinary tract and the female urinary tract. Although a broad spectrum of urologic diseases is encountered daily in clinical practice, considerable effort is directed toward the medical and surgical treatment of voiding disorders. This chapter explains several common urologic procedures such as urethral catheterization, percutaneous suprapubic cystostomy, retrograde urethrography, penile nerve block, and dorsal slit.

A. URETHRAL CATHETERIZATION

1. Indications:
   a. Therapeutic
      - Urinary retention
      - Urinary output monitoring
      - Evacuation of blood clots
      - Intravesical chemotherapy
      - Postoperative urethral stenting
   b. Diagnostic
      - Collection of urine for culture
      - Measurement of the postvoid residual urine
      - Retrograde instillation of contrast agents (cystourethrography)
      - Urodynamic studies

2. Contraindications:
    a. Acute prostatitis
    b. Suspected urethral disruption associated with blunt or pene-
       trating trauma
        • Blood at urethral meatus
        • Hemiscrotum
        • Perineal ecchymoses
        • Nonpalpable prostate
        • Inability to void
    c. Severe urethral stricture

3. Anesthesia:
    Recommend 2% lidocaine jelly

4. Equipment:
    a. Urethral catheterization kit (includes Foley catheter, povi-
       done-iodine solution, lubricating jelly, 10-ml syringe with
       sterile normal saline, gloves, sterile towels, and urinary
       drainage bag)
    b. Recommend 18F Foley catheter for male and 16F for female
       patients
    c. Recommend 22F–24F Foley catheter for blood clot irrigation

5. Positioning:
    Supine (men), frog-leg (women)

6. Technique—Catheterization of Men:
    a. Place sterile towels around the penis (see Figure 7.1).
    b. Test the balloon of the catheter, lubricate the catheter with
       lubricating jelly, and set it aside on the sterile field.
    c. Retract the foreskin (if present). Grasp the penis laterally
       with the nondominant hand and place it on maximum
       stretch perpendicular to the body to straighten the anterior
       urethra.
    d. Swab the glans with povidone-iodine with the dominant
       hand. Observe sterile technique at all times.
    e. Inject 10 ml of 2% lidocaine jelly into urethra. Place a sterile
       urethral clamp for 5 minutes to provide anesthesia as well as
       additional lubrication. If lidocaine jelly is not available, it is
       helpful to inject 10 ml of lubricating jelly into the urethra.

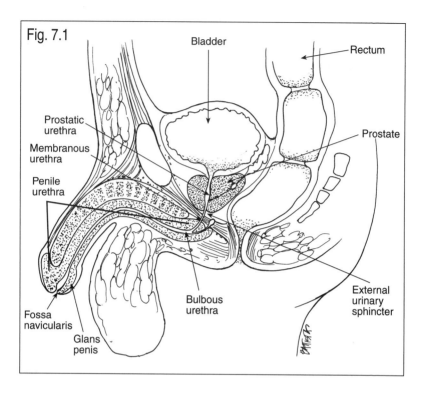

Fig. 7.1

f. Grasp the catheter with the dominant hand. (see Figure 7.2)
g. Using steady, gentle pressure, advance the catheter into the urethra until both the hub of the catheter is reached and urine is returned. Inflate the balloon with 10 ml normal saline.
h. If urine is not returned, irrigate the catheter to confirm correct placement prior to inflating the balloon.
i. Replace the foreskin to prevent a paraphimosis. Connect the catheter to a urinary drainage bag.
j. If the catheter cannot easily be passed, a strategy for successful catheterization must be planned.

7. Strategies for Difficult Catheterization of Men

If resistance is met during catheter advancement, manually palpate the catheter tip to define the point of obstruction along the urethra (see Figure 7.3). Once the location and nature of the lesion is defined, the next step is to develop a strategy for bypassing the obstruction.

a. Anterior urethral obstruction—urethral stricture, a concen-

Fig. 7.2

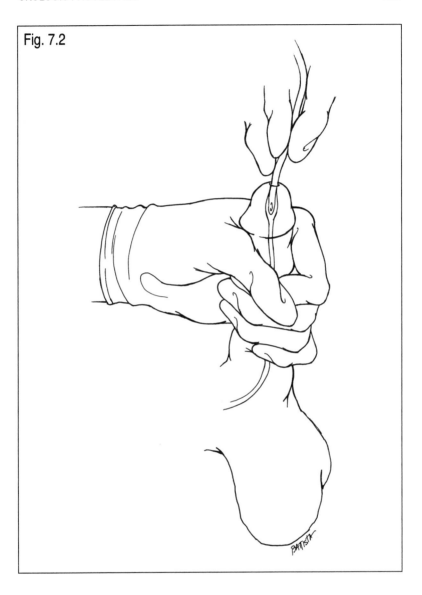

tric narrowing of the lumen by scar tissue. Can occur at
the fossa navicularis, bulbous urethra, or along the penile
urethra.
- Etiology: sexually transmitted disease, prior urethral
  instrumentation including transurethral resection of
  prostate (TURP), trauma.
- Signs/symptoms: splayed and/or slow stream, straining.

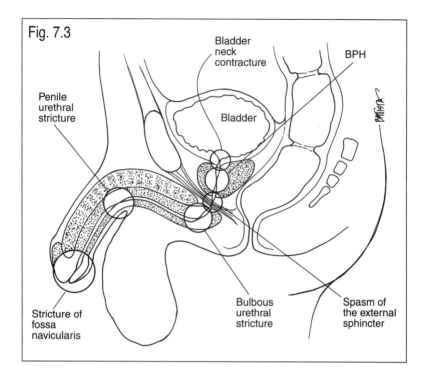

Fig. 7.3

- Strategy for penile urethral stricture:
  (1) Use 16F or smaller straight-tip Foley catheter.
  (2) If unsuccessful, consult urology department to attempt catheter placement.
- Strategy for bulbous urethral stricture:
  (1) Same as above.
  (2) If unsuccessful, 16F coudé-tip catheter will better negotiate the natural angle of the bulbomembranous junction. A coudé catheter has a curved tip that enables one to better engage the normal S-shaped curve of the bulbomembranous junction or to bypass an enlarged, obstructing prostate in the male urethra. To insert a coudé catheter, always keep the angled tip pointing superiorly and follow steps 6a–6j.
  b. Posterior urethral obstructions
- Spasm of the external urinary sphincter
  (1) Etiology: contraction of the voluntary sphincter secondary to anxiety or pain. Often the cause of unsuccessful catheterization of men < 50 years old.
  (2) Signs: As the catheter tip approaches the sphincter, the patient becomes tense and complains of pain.

(3) Strategy: (a) Inject 10 ml of lubricant (water-soluble jelly works as well as 2% lidocaine jelly). (b) After reaching the sphincter, pull the catheter back a few centimeters. (c) Distract the patient with conversation and by having him breathe deeply. (d) Advance the Foley catheter steadily with a slow, gentle pressure when the patient is relaxed.

- Benign prostatic hypertrophy (BPH)
  (1) Suspect with age >60 years, prior transurethral resection of the prostate (TURP), treatment with finasteride (Proscar), terazosin (Hytrin), doxazosin (Cardura), or tamsulosin (Flomax).
  (2) Symptoms: hesitancy, intermittent and/or slow stream, straining, sensation of incomplete emptying.
  (3) Strategy: (a) A large catheter (18F or 20F) provides the additional stiffness needed to overcome the obstruction. A coudé-tip catheter is often helpful for negotiating the angle between the bulbous and membranous urethra (see Figure 7.1). (b) Use the two-person technique: While catheter placement is attempted in the usual fashion, the assistant places a lubricated index finger in the rectum and palpates the apex of the prostate. The tip of the catheter usually can be felt just distal to the apex (see Figure 7.4). The index finger presses anteriorly, thus elevating the apex and straightening out the area of obstruction (see Figure 7.5).
- Prostate cancer: typically is not the sole cause of difficult catheterization unless the cancer is locally advanced. Strategy is similar to that for BPH.
- Bladder neck contracture.
  (1) Etiology: prior open or radical retropubic prostatectomy, bladder neck incision, or TURP.
  (2) Symptoms: hesitancy, intermittent and/or slow stream, straining, sensation of incomplete emptying.
  (3) Strategy: (a) Attempt a 12F coudé catheter placement, following steps 6a–6j. (b) Consult urology department.

8. Technique—Catheterization of Women:

a. Place patient in a frog-leg position (see Figure 7.6). Alternatively, for women who are unable to abduct the thighs, flexion at the hips provides easy access to the urethra.
b. Adequate lighting is essential.

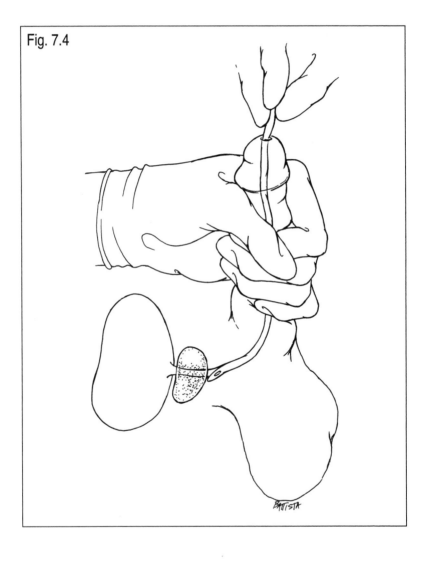

Fig. 7.4

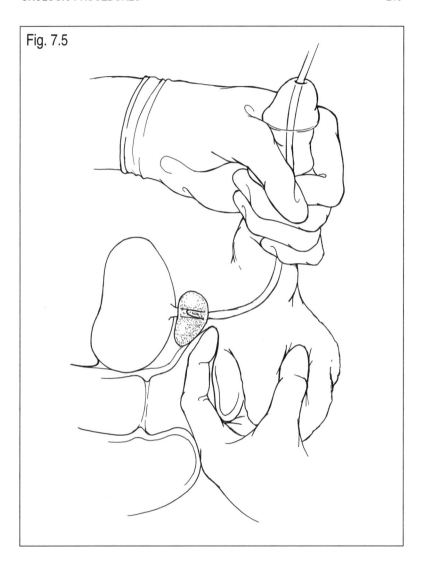

Fig. 7.5

c. Place sterile towels around the introitus.
d. Use the nondominant hand to spread apart labia minora (see Figure 7.7).
e. With good lighting, visualize urethral meatus.
f. Use the dominant hand to swab the urethral meatus with providone-iodine solution.
g. Using sterile technique, grasp a lubricated 16F catheter with the dominant hand and advance it approximately 10 cm through the urethral meatus or until urine is returned.

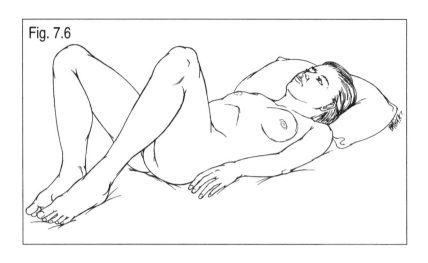

Fig. 7.6

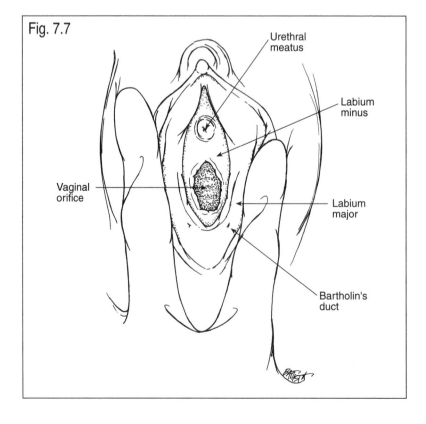

Fig. 7.7

Urethral meatus

Labium minus

Vaginal orifice

Labium major

Bartholin's duct

h. Inflate the balloon with 10 ml normal saline.

i. Attach the catheter to the urinary drainage bag.

j. If the urethral meatus cannot be easily located, place the patient in the dorsal lithotomy position.

k. The urethral meatus may still be difficult to visualize due to vaginal atrophy, congenital female hypospadias, or a prior surgical procedure that has altered the location of the meatus. In these instances, the meatus is typically located deeper within the vaginal vault and anteriorly in the urethrovaginal septum.

l. A vaginal speculum may be helpful for locating the meatus.

m. Confirmation of the correct catheter position can be accomplished by placing a lubricated index finger in the vagina and palpating the catheter anteriorly through the urethrovaginal septum.

9. Complications and Management:

a. Suspicion of false passage
  • Best evaluated by cystoscopy.
  • Abort further attempts and consult urology department.

b. Relief of acute retention: It is usually safe to drain the entire bladder contents rapidly. Observe the patient for postobstructive diuresis. If the urine output is >200 ml/hr over the next several hours or if the patient has other comorbid diseases (i.e., congestive heart failure, azotemia, sepsis), then consider a hospital admission.

c. Hypotension
  • Early hypotension is typically a vasovagal response to the acute relief of a distended bladder.
  • Late hypotension can occur from excessive postobstructive diuresis.

d. Hematuria
  • Caused by traumatic catheter placement or by small mucosal disruptions following the acute relief of a distended bladder.
  • Treat with fluids, catheter irrigation, and monitoring.

e. Paraphimosis
  • See Section E in this chapter for treatment.

B. PERCUTANEOUS SUPRAPUBIC CYSTOSTOMY

Two main types of percutaneous suprapubic catheters are the Bonanno percutaneous suprapubic catheter set (Becton–Dickinson and Co., Franklin Lakes, NJ) and Stamey percutaneous suprapubic catheter set in 10F, 12F, or 14F (Cook Urological, Spencer, IA).

1. Indications:

    a. Urethral stricture
    b. False passage
    c. Inability to catheterize
    d. Acute prostatitis
    e. Traumatic urethral disruption
    f. Periurethral abscess

2. Contraindications:

    a. Prior midline infraumbilical incision
    b. Nondistended bladder
    c. Coagulopathy
    d. Pregnancy
    e. Carcinoma of the bladder
    f. Pelvic irradiation

3. Anesthesia:

    1% lidocaine

4. Equipment:

    a. Bonanno percutaneous suprapubic catheter set or Stamey percutaneous suprapubic catheter set in 10F, 12F, or 14F
    b. Urinary drainage bag
    c. Sterile prep solution
    d. Sterile gloves and towels
    e. 20-gauge spinal needle
    f. 10-ml syringe (two)
    g. 1% lidocaine
    h. 22- to 25-gauge needles
    i. 3-0 nylon suture
    j. Needle driver
    k. Suture scissors
    l. Scalpel

5. Positioning:

    Supine

6. Technique:

   a. Administer appropriate antibiotics, especially if urinary tract infection is suspected.
   b. Percuss the suprapubic area to confirm an adequately distended bladder.
   c. Shave, prep, and drape the suprapubic area.
   d. Assemble the catheter.

   For the Bonanno catheter: Place the disposable catheter sleeve adjacent to the suture disc (see Figure 7.8). Insert the 18-gauge

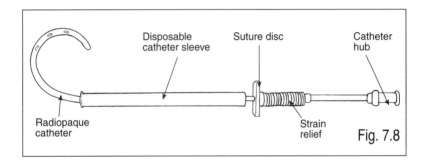

Fig. 7.8

puncture needle into the catheter so that the needle tip is always directed along the inside of the curve. To prevent the needle tip from damaging the inside of the catheter during assembly, advance the needle and the catheter sleeve simultaneously (the catheter sleeve straightens the J of the distal catheter), always maintaining the needle tip within the center of the catheter sleeve (see Figure 7.9). Once the bevel of the needle extends beyond the

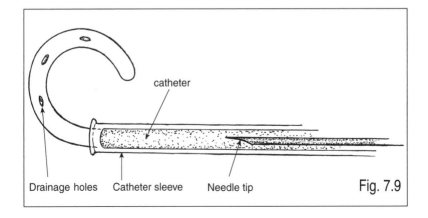

Fig. 7.9

end of the catheter, remove the disposable catheter sleeve and rotate the pink needle hub clockwise to lock the needle to the catheter hub.

For the Stamey catheter: Guide the needle obturator into the catheter tip to stretch and straighten the self-retaining mechanism of the Malecot catheter. Secure its position with the Luer lock to close the Malecot wings (see Figure 7.10).

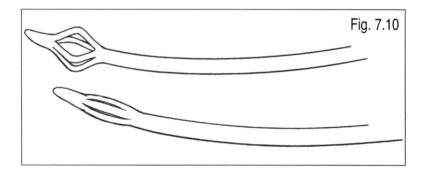

Fig. 7.10

e. If catheter damage occurs during assembly, discard the catheter.
f. Anesthetize the skin with 1% lidocaine at a point 4 cm above the symphysis pubis in the midline (see Figure 7.11). If the patient has a previous midline incision scar, anesthetize 4 cm above the symphysis pubis and 2 cm lateral to the incision. Direct the angle of the needle inferomedially toward the symphysis. Real-time ultrasonography can be helpful.
g. Insert the spinal needle into the anesthetized skin 4 cm above the pubic symphysis in the midline (also 2 cm lateral to the midline if an old midline incision scar is present). Direct the needle toward the symphysis, using a 60° angle to the skin (see Figure 7.12). After the skin is punctured, two additional points of resistance (rectus fascia and bladder wall) are encountered as the needle is advanced. Stop needle advancement after penetrating through the second point of resistance.
h. Remove the obturator of the spinal needle and attach a 10-ml syringe.
i. If urine is not aspirated, the obturator of the spinal needle can be safely replaced and the needle can be advanced up to 1 cm at a time until urine is aspirated.
j. If urine is aspirated, leave the needle in place as a guide.

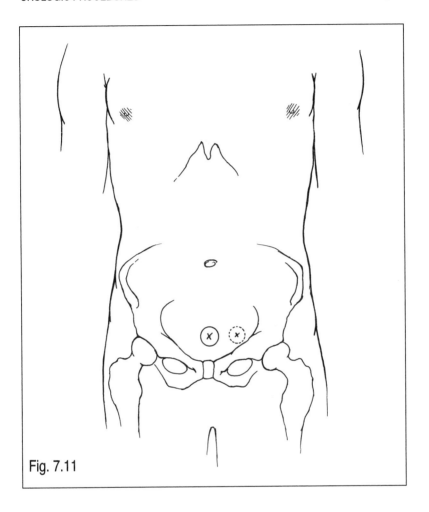

Fig. 7.11

k. If the catheter is larger than 14F, consider making a small stab wound on the puncture site with a scalpel to aid catheter insertion. Next, take the previously assembled suprapubic catheter and puncture the skin adjacent to the spinal needle. Advance the suprapubic catheter in a similar manner as described above (step g), following the tract of the spinal needle. The catheter has a reference mark on the needle obturator indicating the distance at which the catheter should have penetrated the bladder in most patients.

l. Remove the black vent plug (for Bonanno catheter), attach a 10-ml syringe to the catheter hub, and aspirate.

m. Caution: Once the needle has been withdrawn from a supra-

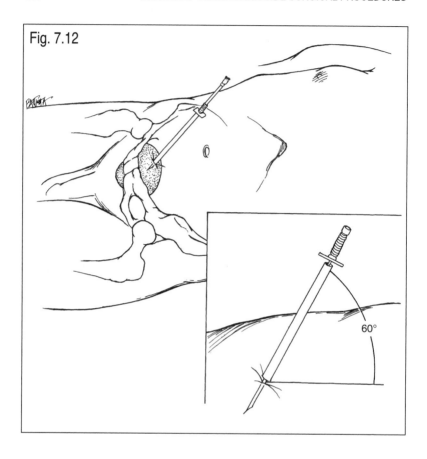

Fig. 7.12

pubic catheter, do not reinsert it! Remove the entire device from the patient and reassemble as in step d.

n. Once urine is obtained, advance the catheter an additional 1–2 cm.

o. Disengage the suprapubic catheter and the needle obturator, and advance the catheter.
   • For the Bonanno catheter: Stabilize the catheter and rotate the pink hub of the needle obturator counterclockwise. Stabilize the needle while advancing the catheter over it until the suture disc lies flush with the skin.
   • For the Stamey catheter: Stabilize the catheter and rotate the white hub of the needle obturator counterclockwise. This maneuver opens the Malecot wings.

p. Aspirate again to confirm proper catheter placement. Insert the connecting tube between the catheter and the urinary drainage bag.

q. For the Stamey catheter, slowly withdraw the catheter until the Malecot wings meet the resistance of the bladder wall. Advance the catheter approximately 2 cm back into the bladder to allow for movement.
r. Secure the catheter to the skin with 3-0 nylon suture. Tape the catheter to the abdominal wall to avoid kinking the tubing.

7. Complications and Management:

a. Bowel injury
- Adequate bladder distention and ultrasonographic guidance are helpful in preventing injury to loops of small bowel.
- If bowel is entered, one may exchange the needle and continue with the procedure. Peritonitis is rare.
b. Hematuria/clots
- Transient hematuria is common, but usually clears quickly.
- If obstruction of the catheter from clots is suspected, gently irrigate the suprapubic catheter with normal saline. These percutaneous cystostomy catheters are of small caliber (14-gauge lumen, Bonanno; 10F–14F, Stamey) and are often insufficient for treating gross hematuria with clot obstruction.
- Leakage around the insertion site may indicate catheter damage, obstruction, or bladder spasm.
- Urology consult.

C. RETROGRADE URETHROGRAPHY

Retrograde urethrogram is the best study for visualizing the anterior male urethra. It is valuable in diagnosing a urethral disruption after a blunt or penetrating trauma to the pelvis and in evaluating many urethral structural abnormalities, such as strictures, diverticula, fistulas, and anterior urethral valves.

1. Indications:

a. Suspected urethral injury after trauma
b. Evaluation of anterior urethral stricture
c. Possible urethral diverticulum

2. Contraindications:

Acute urethritis

3. Anesthesia:

None

4. Equipment:

a. Urethral catheterization kit (includes Foley catheter, povidone-iodine solution, lubricating jelly, 10-ml syringe with sterile normal saline, gloves, sterile towels, and urinary drainage bag)
b. Water-soluble contrast agent
c. Catheter-tip syringe
d. Fluoroscopy or radiography equipment

5. Positioning:

Supine for catheter insertion, lateral decubitus for radiographs

6. Technique:

a. Place sterile towels around the penis.
b. Test the balloon of the catheter, lubricate the catheter with lubricating jelly, and set it aside on the sterile field.
c. Retract the foreskin (if present). Grasp the penis laterally with the nondominant hand and place it on moderate stretch perpendicular to the body.
d. Swab the glans with povidone-iodine with the dominant hand. Observe sterile technique at all times.
e. Lubricate the catheter with lubricating jelly and grasp with the dominant hand.
f. Using steady, gentle pressure, advance the catheter until the balloon is inserted 2–3 cm into the fossa navicularis (see Figure 7.13).
g. Gently inflate the balloon with 1–2 ml normal saline until it tamponades the urethral lumen.
h. Inject 10–15 ml of water-soluble contrast agent, and obtain appropriate radiographs.
i. Caution: Avoid excessive force or overdistension of the urethra to prevent contrast extravasation to the corpus spongiosum or penile vasculature.
j. After confirming a satisfactory radiographic evaluation of the urethra, deflate the balloon and remove the catheter.
k. Replace the foreskin to prevent a paraphimosis.
l. If complete urethral stricture or severe urethral disruption is

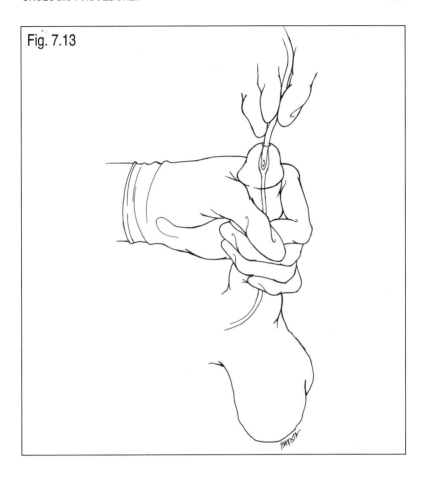

Fig. 7.13

confirmed, consider placing a percutaneous suprapubic cystostomy (see section B in this chapter).

D. PENILE NERVE BLOCK

1. Indications:
   a. Reduction of paraphimosis
   b. Circumcision
   c. Dorsal slit
   d. Repair of penile trauma

2. Contraindications:
   Noncorrectable coagulopathy

3. Anesthesia:

   1% lidocaine solution; avoid epinephrine

4. Equipment:
   a. Sterile prep solution
   b. Sterile gloves and towels
   c. 10-ml syringe
   d. 22-gauge needle

5. Positioning:

   Supine

6. Technique:
   a. Prep and drape the suprapubic skin, penis, and anterolateral scrotum.
   b. Identify the penopubic junction.
   c. Using a 22-gauge needle on a syringe filled with 1% plain lidocaine, puncture the skin 1 cm cranial to the penopubic junction near the lateral border of the penis on the patient's right side (see Figure 7.14).
   d. Advance the needle until the needle tip penetrates through the subtle resistance of Buck's fascia.
   e. Gently aspirate to prevent intravascular injection prior to injecting 5 ml 1% plain lidocaine just beneath Buck's fascia (see Figure 7.15).

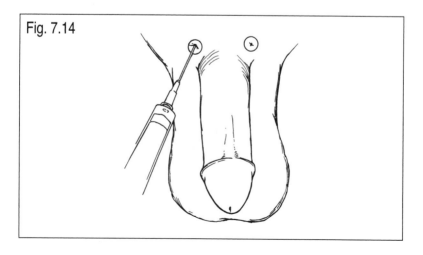

Fig. 7.14

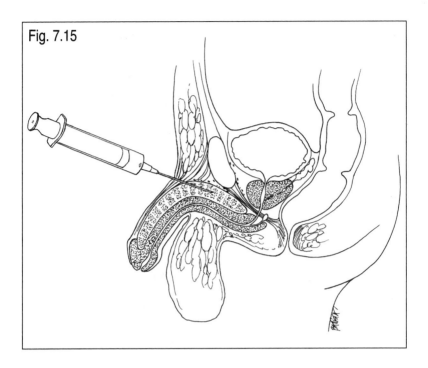

Fig. 7.15

f. Repeat the same sequence on the patient's left side (see Figure 7.14).
g. At the base of the penis, circumferentially infiltrate the skin with approximately 5 ml 1% lidocaine. Care must be taken to avoid puncturing the superficial dorsal veins of the penis and their tributaries.
h. Wait at least 5 minutes to obtain an adequate penile block.

7. Complications and Management:
   a. Expanding hematoma: Apply direct pressure to control hemorrhage.
   b. Penile ischemia: Avoid premixed local anesthetics containing epinephrine.

E. DORSAL SLIT

Phimosis is the condition in which the foreskin cannot be retracted over the glans due to constriction of the orifice, usually from repeated episodes of balanitis. Paraphimosis is the condition in which the foreskin, once retracted proximal to the glans, cannot be replaced to its normal position. The foreskin is edematous and tender with paraphimosis. With an adequate penile block, paraphimosis can be manually reduced in most circumstances by compressing the glans with gentle, steady pressure for 5–10 minutes to reduce the edema, followed by pulling the foreskin over the glans with the two-handed technique (see Figure 7.16).

Fig. 7.16

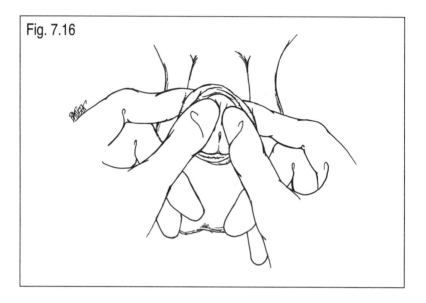

Additionally, a dorsal slit can be performed for severe phimosis or unreducible paraphimosis.

1. Indications:
   a. Unreducible paraphimosis
   b. Severe phimosis associated with acute or recurrent infections (balanitis, urethritis)
   c. Voiding difficulty or inability to catheterize

2. Contraindications:
   a. Noncorrectable coagulopathy
   b. Hypospadias

3. Anesthesia:
   Penile block

4. Equipment:
   a. Sterile prep solution
   b. Sterile gloves and towels
   c. Two straight clamps
   d. Scissors
   e. Needle driver
   f. 4-0 chromic sutures
   g. 10-ml syringe
   h. 22-gauge needle
   i. 1% lidocaine

5. Positioning:

   Supine

6. Technique:
   a. Administer antibiotics if infection is present.
   b. Sterile prep and drape penis, presymphysis, and anterior scrotum. Be sure to adequately prep beneath foreskin.
   c. Place penile block (see section D).
   d. Place a straight clamp across the dorsal surface of the foreskin in the midline, carefully avoiding injury to the glans (see Figure 7.17). The tip of the clamp must be placed 0.5–1 cm proximal to the corona on the mucosal (inner) surface.
   e. After clamping for 1 minute, remove the clamp and cut along the crimp mark. Adequate length of incision is confirmed by the ability of the foreskin to easily retract over the glans.
   f. Suture both sides with running 4-0 chromic suture beginning at the apex of the incision and progressing toward the distal foreskin (see Figure 7.18). Both the mucosal (inner) and serosal (outer) skin edges must always be visualized and incorporated into the closure when suturing the wound.
   g. Dress with sterile gauze.

7. Complications and Management:
   a. Bleeding
      • The crushing straight clamp should minimize bleeding during the procedure.
      • Apply direct pressure on any bleeding point and oversew if necessary.
      • If bleeding persists, an Elastoplast dressing should

Fig. 7.17

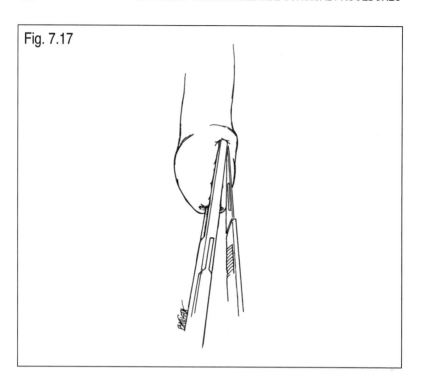

Fig. 7.18

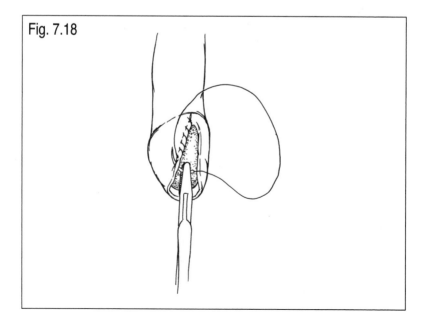

tamponade it. To minimize distal glandular ischemia, do not apply the dressing too tightly.
  b. Infection
    • Local wound care
    • Antibiotics
  c. Injuries to the urethra or the glans
    • Urology consult

II. GYNECOLOGY

Gynecology involves the evaluation and treatment of various disorders and diseases of the female reproductive tract, as well as its normal physiological function. Culdocentesis and surgical drainage of a Bartholin abscess are two common bedside procedures performed in clinical practice.

A. CULDOCENTESIS

1. Indications:
    a. Suspected pelvic abscess
    b. Possible ruptured ectopic pregnancy

2. Contraindications:
    a. Obliterated cul-de-sac
    b. Severely retroverted uterus

3. Anesthesia:
    2% lidocaine jelly, 1% lidocaine solution

4. Equipment:
    a. Sterile prep solution
    b. Gloves
    c. Speculum
    d. Single-tooth tenaculum or sponge forceps
    e. 10-ml syringe (two)
    f. 20- or 22-gauge spinal needle
    g. Long cotton-tip swabs
    h. Kelly clamp
    i. Scalpel on long handle

5. Positioning:

   Dorsal lithotomy

6. Technique:

   a. Swab the introitus with sterile prep solution.
   b. Insert the speculum. If the posterior cul-de-sac is not fully
      prepared, use the long cotton-tip swabs to complete the
      prep. The posterior cul-de-sac will be bulging or tender if an
      abscess is present (see Figure 7.19).

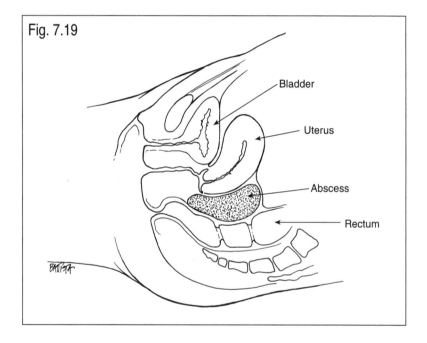

Fig. 7.19

   c. Place a long cotton-tip swab generously lubricated with 2%
      lidocaine jelly on the midline posterior vaginal wall 2 cm be-
      low the cervix. Wait a few minutes for adequate anesthesia.
   d. The posterior lip of the cervix can be gently grasped with a
      sponge forceps and elevated. Alternatively, infiltrate the pos-
      terior cervical lip with 2–3 ml of 1% lidocaine, and once anes-
      thetized, cautiously apply a single-tooth tenaculum. Elevate
      the cervix (see Figure 7.20).
   e. With the spinal needle mounted on the 10-ml syringe, insert
      the needle tip through the anesthetized midline posterior
      vaginal wall into the cul-de-sac and aspirate (see Figure 7.21).

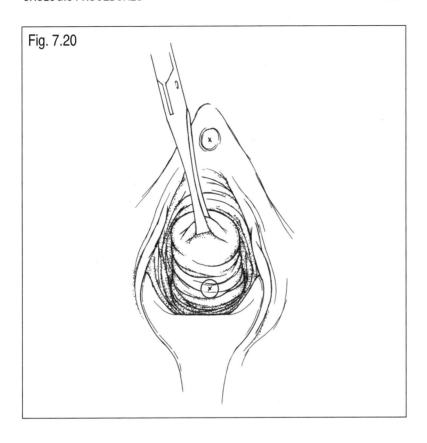

Fig. 7.20

f. The presence of blood or pus confirms the diagnosis. If fluid cannot be withdrawn, reposition the needle. Send fluid for culture and/or analysis as indicated.

g. If an abscess (pus) is encountered, it must be fully incised and drained. Incise the vaginal mucosa at the puncture site with a #15 or #11 scalpel.

h. Bluntly spread with a Kelly clamp and express the pus (see Figure 7.22).

i. Irrigate until the abscess cavity is clear.

j. If no fluid is aspirated, it is difficult to unequivocally rule out an abscess or fluid collection in the cul-de-sac. Sonography can be helpful in select cases.

7. Complications and Management:

Bleeding: Apply direct pressure on the bleeding site with the long cotton-tip swab.

Fig. 7.21

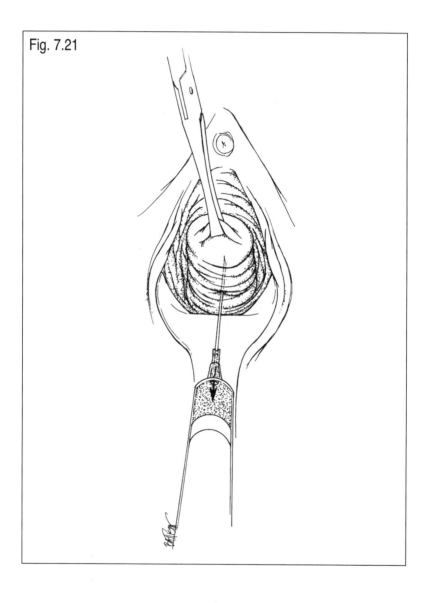

Fig. 7.22

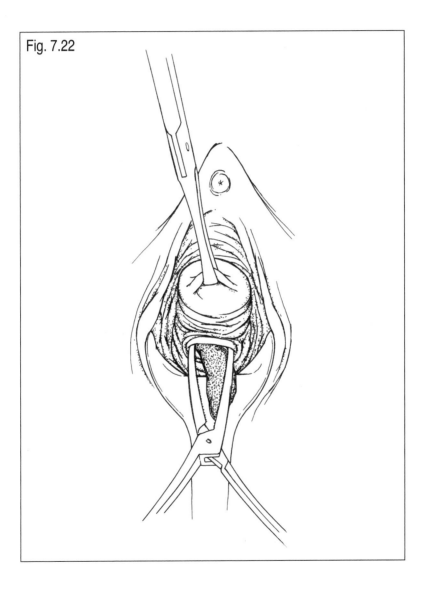

B. INCISION AND DRAINAGE OF BARTHOLIN ABSCESS

A Bartholin cyst results from a cystic dilation of the duct after blockage of the duct orifice and presents as a unilateral swelling lateral to the posterior fourchette. Bartholin cysts are usually 1–3 cm in diameter and are asymptomatic. However, these cysts can become quite painful if secondarily infected.

1. Indications:
   a. Relief of symptoms
   b. Failure of conservative medical management

2. Contraindications:
   a. Nonfluctuant cyst/abscess
   b. Diabetic patient with the susceptibility to necrotizing infection

3. Anesthesia:
   1% lidocaine solution

4. Equipment:
   a. Sterile prep solution
   b. Sterile towels and gloves
   c. #15 scalpel
   d. Kelly clamp
   e. 10-ml syringe
   f. Word Bartholin Gland catheter (Rusch Corporation, Duluth, GA)
   g. Saline irrigation
   h. Nu Gauze packing
   i. 22- to 25-gauge needles

5. Positioning:
   Dorsal lithotomy

6. Technique:
   a. Administer broad-spectrum antibiotics. Use analgesics as necessary.
   b. Examination should reveal a fluctuant, ripened abscess. Prep and drape.

   c. If the cyst is not yet fluctuant, management consists of sitz
      baths, antibiotics, and analgesics. Drainage is indicated when
      fluctuant.
   d. Carefully inject 1% lidocaine circumferentially around the
      abscess while aspirating intermittently to prevent intravas-
      cular or intra-abscess injection.
   e. The abscess is approached medially through the mucosa of
      the vagina. A 1- to 2-cm incision through the vaginal mucosa
      into the abscess cavity is sufficient for drainage (see Figure
      7.23).

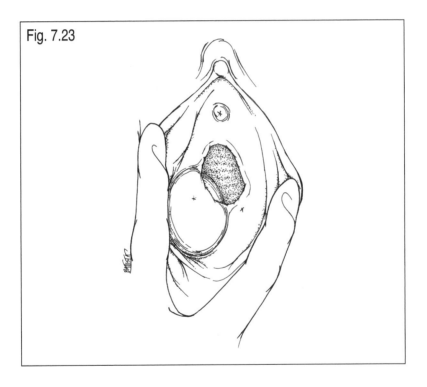

Fig. 7.23

   f. Send fluid for culture, including tests for gonococcal and
      chlamydial infections.
   g. Manually (or with a Kelly clamp) express all of the pus and
      break up loculations.
   h. Copiously irrigate the abscess cavity with normal saline.
      Pack the cavity with Nu Gauze dressing.
   i. Alternatively, a Word Bartholin Gland catheter may be used.
      This is a 5-cm, 10F rubber catheter with an inflatable balloon
      tip. The catheter tip is inserted through a 1- to 2-mm stab in-

cision into the abscess cavity after it has been irrigated. Inflate the 5-ml balloon with normal saline and tuck up the free end of the catheter into the vagina. The catheter is left in place for up to 4 weeks to allow complete epithelialization of the new tract.

7. Complications and Management:
a. Bleeding
   - Apply direct pressure.
   - If not successful, packing the cavity with Nu Gauze should stop the bleeding.
b. Recurrence
   - Should be avoidable by initially providing complete drainage of the abscess, followed by daily packing changes.
   - Elective operative marsupialization should prevent recurrence.

CHAPTER 8

PLASTIC SURGERY AND HAND PROCEDURES

Author: Gregory M. Galdino, M.D.

PLASTIC SURGERY AND HAND PROCEDURES

The specialty of plastic surgery encompasses a wide variety of surgical challenges, from managing the most difficult of wounds, to repairing vascular, tendon, and nerve injuries. It is unique in that the aesthetic outcome is of paramount concern, in concert with restoration of function, form, and continuity. Plastic surgery requires a broad base of skills, including identifying important anatomical structures, inducing regional anesthesia, and managing difficult wounds of the face and hand.

I. REGIONAL ANESTHESIA

Local anesthetics work by producing nerve conduction blockade at the level of nerve membrane receptors. The most commonly used agent is lidocaine. Addition of epinephrine (epi) reduces bleeding and systemic absorption by local vasoconstriction. The toxic limit of lidocaine is 5 mg/kg without epinephrine and 7 mg/kg with epinephrine (Note: 1% lidocaine contains 10 mg/ml). Properties of common local anesthetics are shown below.

A. LOCAL/FIELD BLOCK

1. Indications:
   a. Anesthesia for surgical procedures
   b. Anesthesia for wounds that require irrigation, debridement, and/or repair

Local Anesthetic	Onset	Maximum dose (mg/kg)		Duration of action (hrs)	
		plain	with epi	plain	with epi
Bupivacaine (Marcaine)	slow	2.5	3.5	2.0–4.0	4.0–8.0
Lidocaine (Xylocaine)	rapid	5.0	7.0	0.5–2.0	1.0–4.0
Procaine (Novocaine)	slow	6.0	9.0	0.25–0.5	0.5–1.0
Tetracaine (Pontocaine)	slow	1.5	2.5	2.0–3.0	2.0–4.0

Topical anesthetics are useful in the pediatric population, but require long application times for dermal anesthesia.

EMLA Cream	Onset, 1–2 hours with occlusive dressing	Duration, 3–4 hours
(Lidocaine 2.5% and Prilocaine 2.5%)		
Maximum recommended application	up to 10 kg	100 cm^2
area:	up to 20 kg	600 cm^2
	above 20 kg	2000 cm^2

Mucosal Topical Anesthetics

Hurricaine and Cetacaine both are applied to the mucosa for anesthesia. They contain benzocaine (20% and 14%, respectively) as the active ingredient. Onset is within minutes. Absorption is related to the length of application. Extended periods of application are to be avoided. Ethyl chloride applied topically may provide brief anesthesia by frosting the skin to reduce discomfort of needle injection for local anesthesia.

2. Contraindications:
   a. None when using local anesthetics without epinephrine.
   b. Epinephrine should not be used at anatomic sites supplied by end-arteries (fingers, toes, nose, ears, penis) or in infection-prone wounds (animal/human bites, contaminated wounds).

3. Anesthesia:
   Choose from the above chart and tailor choice to individual patient based on the duration of procedure; time to onset; and location, type, and extent of wound. Long-and short-acting anesthetics can be mixed in a 50:50 ratio to achieve benefits of both.

4. Equipment:

a. Sterile prep solution
b. Sterile gloves and towels
c. 25-gauge needle
d. 10-ml syringe

5. Positioning:

Varies with location of wound

6. Technique:

a. Sterile prep wound with antiseptic such as Betadine, cleanse with alcohol swab.
b. Stretch skin taut to facilitate penetration, and directly infiltrate local anesthetic through wound edges and inside wound with a long 25-gauge needle; minimize needle sticks by orienting needle longitudinally along axis of wound and injecting beneath skin edges (see Figure 8.1).
c. Inject the anesthetic slowly or add $NaHCO_3$ (1 ml 10% $NaHCO_3$ to 9 ml 1% lidocaine) to reduce pain on infiltration. If more $NaHCO_3$ is added, it will precipitate in the lidocaine. If this occurs, do not use the solution.
d. Irrigate wound thoroughly with normal saline; use an 18-gauge needle to introduce holes in the top of a plastic saline bottle and use this as a squirt bottle to irrigate.
e. Sterilely drape the wound.

7. Complications and Management:

a. Intravascular injection or overdose
   • Initial signs of toxicity include dizziness, restlessness, paresthesias, and twitching, and may lead to generalized seizures, hypotension, bradycardia, and cardiovascular collapse. Complications are generally self-limited but may require supportive care until effects wear off.
   • Stop the local anesthetic and hyperventilate with 100% O_2.
   • Use IV diazepam (0.1–0.3 mg/kg) for seizures.
   • Initiate ACLS protocols if necessary. Trendelenburg for hypotension and bradycardia. Prolonged CPR is indicated because the effects of the anesthetic will subside as the drug redistributes.

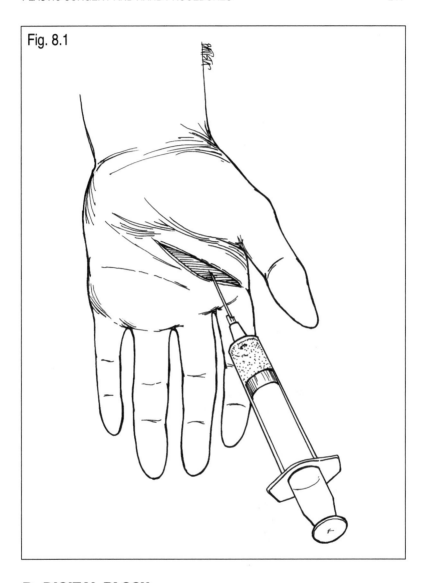

Fig. 8.1

B. DIGITAL BLOCK

1. Indications:

Wounds involving the fingers or thumb

2. Contraindications:

Injury to the digital neurovascular bundle. Perform a thorough neurological examination to the injured area before anesthesia.

3. Anesthesia:

Agents that lack epinephrine (see chart in section A)

4. Equipment:

a. Sterile prep solution
b. Sterile gloves and towels
c. 3/4-inch 25-gauge needle
d. 10-ml syringe

5. Positioning:

Supine with arm extended out on an arm board, palm down

6. Technique:

a. Sterile prep and drape fingers and web spaces.
b. Using a 3/4-inch 25-gauge needle, puncture the skin in the two surrounding interdigital web spaces and advance the needle perpendicular to the horizontal plane of the hand and fingers, with the plunger end of syringe tilted slightly away from distal hand (see Figure 8.2).
c. With the full length of the needle in the web space, aspirate to make sure needle is not intravascular . Inject each of the two surrounding interdigital web spaces with 3 ml of 1% lidocaine, filling them with anesthetic (see Figure 8.3).
d. The digital nerves are located toward the volar surface of the hand, so the needle must be aimed more volarly as well. This is especially true in the thumb.
e. Infiltrate another 3 ml 1% lidocaine at the dorsum of the metacarpophalangeal joint (knuckle) to block the dorsal branches of the radial digital nerve. Avoid circumferential block at base.
f. Allow at least 5 minutes for the onset of anesthesia, depending on the agent. If a total block is not achieved in about 20–30 minutes, then an additional 2 ml may be administered in each web space.

7. Complications and Management:

See section I A 7.

C. WRIST BLOCK

1. Indications:

Complex hand wounds

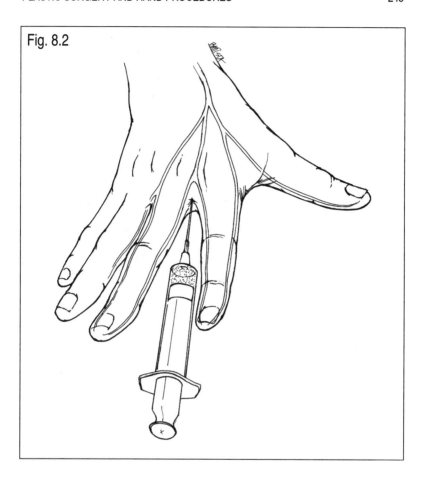

Fig. 8.2

2. Contraindications:

Injury to median/radial/ulnar nerves and vessels. Perform thorough neurological examination before performing block.

3. Anesthesia:

See chart in section A. Recommend 2% lidocaine.

4. Equipment:

a. Sterile prep solution
b. Sterile gloves and towels
c. 25-gauge needle
d. 10-ml syringe

Fig. 8.3

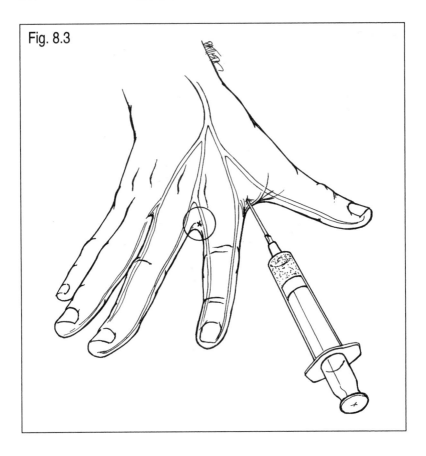

5. Positioning:

   Supine with arm extended out on arm board

6. Technique:

   a. Sterile prep and drape wrist and hand.
   b. Using a 25-gauge needle, inject each of the following four
      sites with 5 ml 2% lidocaine. Be careful not to elicit paresthe-
      sias. Always aspirate before injection to avoid intravascular
      injection.
      • Median nerve: Locate palmaris longus by thumb–5th
        finger opposition and wrist flexion. Inject anesthetic radial
        to palmaris longus at the level of the wrist flexion crease.
      • Ulnar nerve: Locate flexor carpi ulnaris by 5th finger
        abduction and wrist flexion. Inject anesthetic radial to
        flexor carpi ulnaris at level of wrist flexion crease (see
        Figure 8.4).

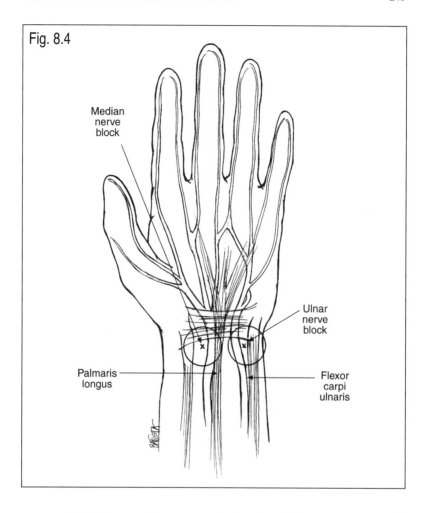

Fig. 8.4

Median nerve block

Ulnar nerve block

Palmaris longus

Flexor carpi ulnaris

- Radial nerve: Accentuate the borders of the anatomic snuff box by thumb abduction. Inject anesthetic over the radial styloid at the base of the snuff box.
- Dorsal cutaneous branch of the ulnar nerve: Inject anesthetic over the ulnar styloid prominence (see Figure 8.5).

7. Complications and Management:
  a. Intravascular injection or overdose
    - See section I A 7.
  b. Paresthesias
    - Stop injection.
    - Advance or pull back needle to move a few millimeters away from nerve aspirate and reinject anesthetic.

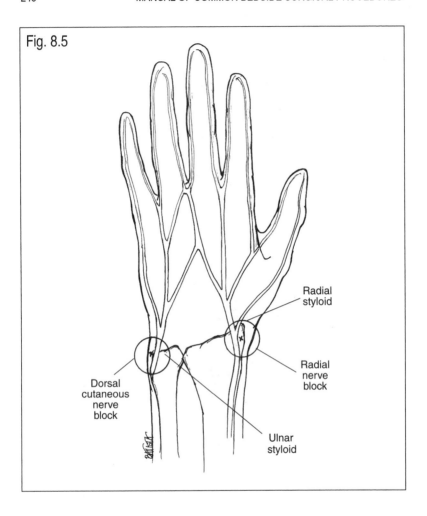

Fig. 8.5

Radial
styloid

Radial
nerve
block

Dorsal
cutaneous
nerve
block

Ulnar
styloid

D. FACIAL BLOCKS

1. Indications:

Extensive wounds involving the forehead, anterior scalp, midface, nose, and upper and lower lips. Distortion from local wound infiltration is minimized with a block, preserving the anatomy for a good aesthetic outcome.

2. Contraindications:

Injury to facial nerves or vessels. Perform thorough neurological examination before performing block.

3. Anesthesia:

See chart in section A. Recommend 1% lidocaine; onset 4–6 minutes.

4. Equipment:

a. Sterile prep solution
b. Sterile gloves and towels
c. 25-gauge needle
d. 10-ml syringe

5. Positioning:

Supine

6. Technique:

a. Sterile prep and drape the injured area of the face and nerve to be blocked.
b. Using a 25-gauge needle, inject each of the following areas specific to the block desired:
    - Forehead block: forehead and anterior scalp, unilateral or bilateral. The supraorbital and supratrochlear nerves supply the forehead and anterior scalp. The supraorbital nerve exits via the supraorbital notch, which can usually be palpated in the supraorbital ridge. The supratrochlear nerve exits just medial to the supraorbital notch. There are two techniques for achieving adequate anesthesia in this area. The techniques and zone of anesthesia (see Figure 8.6).
        (1) Inject 3–5 ml over the supraorbital notch while directing some anesthetic medially.
        (2) Inject a continuous subcutaneous tract of anesthetic along the brow line from midline (if anesthetizing only one side) to the lateral orbital rim.
    - Infraorbital block: upper lip, lateral-inferior nose, lower eyelid. The infraorbital nerve can be approached intraorally or externally through the skin. The infraorbital foramen lies approximately 1.5 cm below the inferior orbital rim in a perpendicular line with the supraorbital notch, nasal portion of the pupil, corner of the mouth, and mental foramen, and 2 cm from the lateral aspect of the nose, as indicated in Figure 8.6. The zone of anesthesia with unilateral or bilateral block also is shown in Figure 8.6.

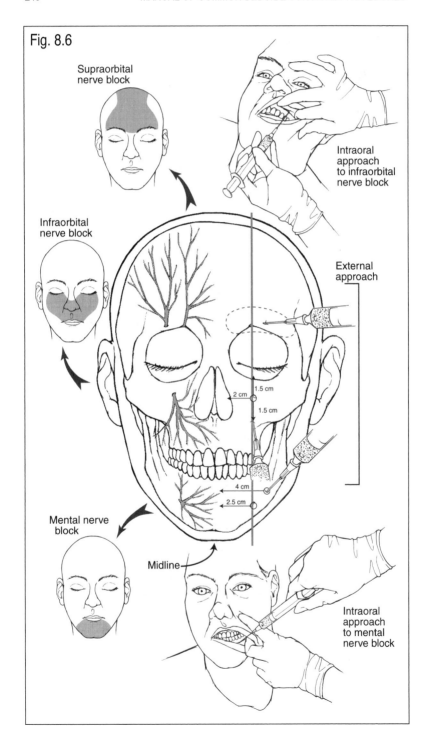

Fig. 8.6

Supraorbital nerve block

Intraoral approach to infraorbital nerve block

Infraorbital nerve block

External approach

2 cm   1.5 cm
        1.5 cm

4 cm
2.5 cm

Mental nerve block

Midline

Intraoral approach to mental nerve block

(1) Intraoral approach: Retract upper lip. Identify maxillary canine. Pretreat injection site with topical anesthetic, if possible (see section A). Introduce needle at anterior margin of maxillary canine into gingival-buccal margin. Advance parallel to maxillary bone to area of infraorbital nerve, and inject 1–2 ml of anesthetic. Avoid injecting directly into foramen as this could cause excess pressure on the nerve. (See Figure 8.6.)

(2) Extraoral approach: Identify position of infraorbital nerve, and enter skin 1.5 cm inferior to this directing needle cephalad and advancing toward the infraorbital foramen. Inject 1–2 ml of anesthetic. (See Figure 8.6.)

- Mental block: lower lip, superior chin. The mental nerve foramen resides just inferior to the second mandibular bicuspid, 2.5 cm from the midline, half way between upper and lower edges of the mandible, and in a straight line with other structures as indicated above under infraorbital block, and as shown in Figure 8.6. The mental nerve can be approached both intraorally and extraorally. The zone of anesthesia is indicated in Figure 8.6.

(1) Intraoral approach: Retract lower lip. Apply topical anesthesia, if possible (see section A). Introduce needle inferior to second bicuspid at gingival–buccal margin. Advance to position of mental nerve, aspirate, and inject 1–2 ml anesthetic. (See Figure 8.6.)

(2) Extraoral approach: Enter skin 4 cm from midline, just superior to position of the mental nerve, and advance toward the mental nerve. Inject 1–2 ml anesthetic over the position of the mental foramen. (See Figure 8.6.)

7. Complications:

See section I A 7.

E. AURICULAR BLOCK

1. Indications:

Extensive wounds of the ear requiring minimal distortion of the tissue of the ear

2. Contraindications:

None

3. Anesthesia:

See chart in section A. No epinephrine. Recommend 1% lidocaine; onset 10–15 minutes.

4. Equipment:

   a. Sterile prep solution
   b. Sterile gloves and towels
   c. 2 1/2-inch 25-gauge needle
   d. 10-ml syringe
   e. Small sterile cup or bowl containing anesthetic

5. Positioning:

Lateral decubitus with injured ear facing up

6. Technique:

The ear receives sensory innervation from multiple branches, including auriculotemporal, greater auricular, and lesser occipital. The vagus also supplies the meatal opening. For this reason, circumferential block must be achieved. Insert the needle below the lobule and advance behind the ear parallel to the bone toward the superior portion of the helix, then withdrawal leaving 3–5 ml of anesthetic in a track. Without removing needle, redirect anteriorly toward the tragus and repeat the above injection. Remove, refill, and inject just behind the superior and posterior portion of the helix, leaving a tract in a similar fashion. Again, without removing the needle, redirect anteriorly toward the tragus and inject in a similar fashion (see Figure 8.7).

7. Complications:

See section I A 7.

II. TOURNIQUETS

Tourniquets provide a bloodless field so that injured structures can be identified safely and uninjured parts can be protected.

A. FINGER TOURNIQUET

1. Indications:

Wounds involving the finger or thumb

Fig. 8.7

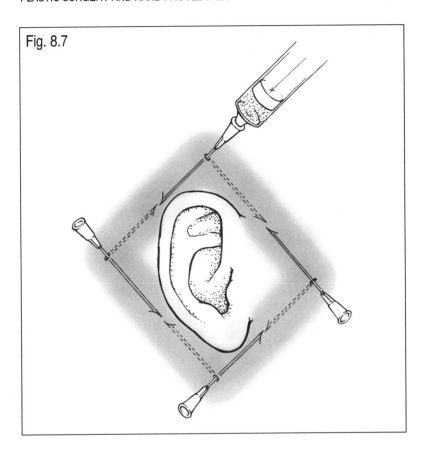

2. Contraindications:

   None

3. Anesthesia:

   Digital block or field block

4. Equipment:

   a. Sterile prep solution
   b. Sterile gloves and towels
   c. 1/4-inch or 1/2-inch sterile Penrose drain
   d. Halsted clamp
   e. Scissors

5. Positioning:

   Supine with arm extended out on arm board

6. Technique:
   a. Sterile prep and drape finger.
   b. Wrap finger tightly with a Penrose drain, starting at fingertip and wrapping down to the base (see Figure 8.8A).
   c. Clamp the Penrose drain to itself at the base of the finger with a Halsted clamp to secure it in place (see Figure 8.8B).

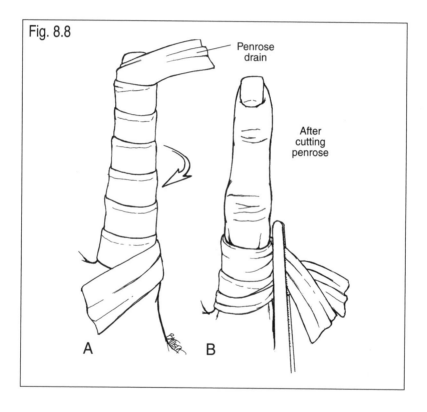

Fig. 8.8

Penrose drain

After cutting penrose

A   B

   d. Cut the Penrose drain distally along finger to expose the wound, leaving it and the Halsted clamp intact at the base of the finger.

7. Complications and Management:
   Ischemia
   • Do not keep the tourniquet on for more than 1 hour.

B. ARM TOURNIQUET

1. Indications:

   Wounds of the forearm and hand

2. Contraindications:

   Previous surgery to the axilla

3. Anesthesia:

   Wrist block or field block

4. Equipment:

   a. Arm tourniquet or blood pressure cuff
   b. 1/2-inch cloth tape
   c. Soft roll cast padding
   d. Ace wrap
   e. Clamps

5. Positioning:

   Supine with arm extended out on arm board

6. Technique:

   a. Place long piece of tape on volar aspect of arm and forearm longitudinally.
   b. Wrap 3–4 layers of cast padding around the arm at the level of the mid-humerus circumferentially.
   c. Place a tourniquet or blood pressure cuff around the cast padding.
   d. To secure the tourniquet's position, lift up distal end of tape, wrap it over the tourniquet, and tape distal end onto proximal end longitudinally.
   e. Hold the patient's hand over his head and exsanguinate the arm by tightly wrapping it with an ace wrap, starting at the fingertips down to level of the tourniquet.
   f. Inflate the tourniquet to 100–150 mm Hg above patient's systolic pressure.
   g. Remove the Ace wrap.
   h. Clamp the tubing to the blood pressure cuff to prevent loss of pressure.

7. Complications and Management:

Ischemia

- Do not keep tourniquet on more than 1 hour; after removal, the forearm needs to be reperfused 5 minutes for each 30 minutes of tourniquet time before reapplication if necessary.
- The arm tourniquet is reasonably comfortable for 15 minutes alone and up to 1 hour when combined with a wrist block.

III. HAND PROCEDURES

Hand injuries account for approximately 20% of all emergency room visits.

A. REMOVAL OF A NAIL

1. Indications:
   a. Nail bed laceration
   b. Inadequately drained subungual hematoma accounting for >25% of the surface area of the nail
   c. Displaced tuft fractures
   d. Extensive paronychia
   e. Complex/crush injury of nail

2. Contraindications:
   None

3. Anesthesia:
   Digital block

4. Equipment:
   a. Sterile prep solution
   b. Sterile gloves and towels
   c. Halsted clamp
   d. Suture and fine scissors

5. Positioning:
   Supine with the hand prone on an arm board

6. Technique:

a. Sterile prep and drape finger and hand.

b. Digital block per section I B.

c. Carefully elevate nail from nail bed using a fine Halsted clamp, without traumatizing the uninjured portions of the nail bed (see Figure 8.9). Alternatively, you can spread fine-tipped scissors just under the nail to aid in elevating the nail from the bed.

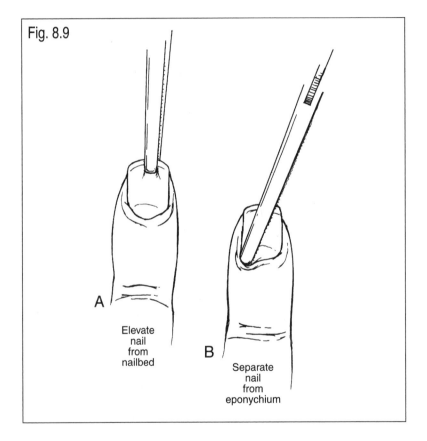

Fig. 8.9

A — Elevate nail from nailbed

B — Separate nail from eponychium

d. Spread fine-tipped scissors under the eponychium to separate the nail from the eponychium. Cut the lateral edges of the eponychium with fine scissors if necessary (see Figure 8.10).

e. Once the nail is free from the nail bed on the deep surface and free from the eponychium on the superficial proximal

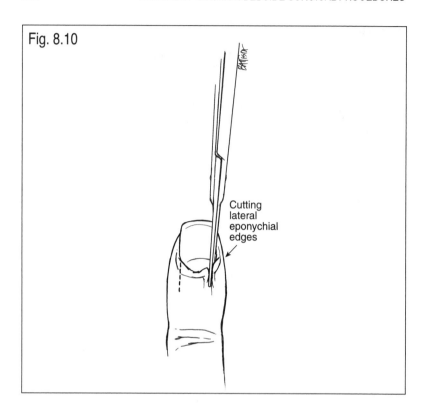

Fig. 8.10

Cutting
lateral
eponychial
edges

surface, remove the nail by grasping the tip of the nail with the clamp and gently pulling the nail straight out.

7. Complications and Management:

Injury to nail bed: Repair per section III B.

B. REPAIR OF NAIL BED LACERATION

1. Indications:

Nail bed laceration

2. Contraindications:

a. Displaced distal phalangeal tuft fracture (50% of all nail bed injuries)
b. Must reduce tuft fracture prior to nail bed repair for normal healing

3. Anesthesia:

   Digital block

4. Equipment:

   a. Sterile prep solution
   b. Sterile gloves and towels
   c. 30-ml syringe
   d. 19-gauge angiographic catheter
   e. Sterile saline
   f. Halsted clamp
   g. Scissors
   h. Needle driver
   i. 18-gauge needle
   j. 6-0 chromic suture on atraumatic needle
   k. 5-0 chromic suture on cutting needle

5. Postioning:

   Supine with arm extended out on arm board and hand prone

6. Technique:

   a. Soak injured finger in dilute Betadine for 5 minutes.
      Sterile prep and drape finger and hand.
   b. Remove nail per section III A.
   c. Irrigate wound with sterile saline using 30-ml syringe with
      19-gauge angiographic catheter. Use about 100 ml saline per
      inch of wound.
   d. Repair the nail bed using simple interrupted 6-0 chromic su-
      tures just deep enough to approximate the surface edges.
      Avoid hitting bone with deep stitches.
   e. If eponychium or paronychium is cut, repair with simple in-
      terrupted 5-0 chromic suture.
   f. Before placement, drill a hole with the 18-gauge needle in
      the center of the intact nail to simplify stitching it in place as
      a splint.
   g. Take the removed intact fingernail, or if the nail is unfit for
      use, an aluminum foil splint (which can be made from suture
      packaging foil), and place it under the eponychial fold in its
      normal anatomic position to provide splinting and protec-
      tion. A 5-0 chromic stay suture can be placed through the
      hole in the nail or splint, then through the nail bed, and back
      through the splint. Slide the splint in place, and then tie the

suture on top of the splint to secure. If a distal tuft fracture is involved, splint as indicated under distal tuft fracture below.

7. Complications and Management:
   a. Infection
      • May need to remove sutures and/or start soaks with saline to promote drainage.
      • Initiate antibiotics if there is surrounding cellulitis.
      • Elevate upper extremity and splint forearm/hand in the position of function. See Chapter 8.

C. DRAINAGE OF SUBUNGAL HEMATOMA

1. Indications:
   Subungual hematoma

2. Contraindications:
   a. Distal phalangeal tuft fracture
   b. Nail bed laceration

3. Anesthesia:
   Digital block

4. Equipment:
   a. Sterile prep solution
   b. Sterile gloves and towels
   c. Either a battery-operated cautery or 18-gauge needle

5. Positioning:
   Supine with arm extended out on arm board and hand prone

6. Technique:
   a. Sterile prep and drape finger and hand.
   b. If there is a nail bed laceration or distal tuft fracture, or if the nail is already broken/dislodged, remove nail per section III A.
   c. If no fracture, pierce the nail over hematoma collection just through the nail with the cautery or needle. Rotate back and

forth to get through the nail when using a needle. Make sure that the hole is large enough to allow postprocedural drainage. Multiple holes may facilitate this (see Figure 8.11).

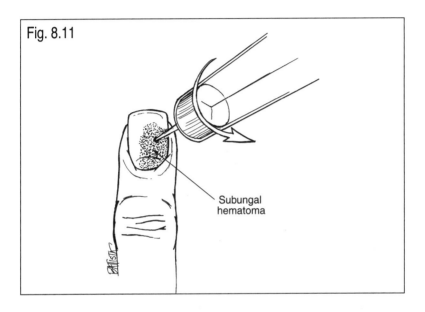

Fig. 8.11

Subungal
hematoma

d. If adequate drainage is achieved, old hematoma will easily escape through the hole as you press down on the nail around the hole.
e. If adequate drainage is not achieved (hematoma covering >25% nail bed area), remove the nail per section III A.

7. Complications and Management:
a. Nail bed injury: Repair per section III B.
b. Inadequate drainage may predispose to infection.

D. TREATMENT OF PARONYCHIA

1. Indications:

Late paronychia (too large to be treated by soaks and antibiotics)

2. Contraindications:

None

3. Anesthesia:

    Digital block

4. Equipment:

    a. Sterile prep solution
    b. Sterile gloves and towels
    c. Halsted clamp
    d. Fine scissors
    e. #15 scalpel blade and handle
    f. Sterile saline
    g. 30-ml syringe
    h. 19-gauge angiocath
    i. Xeroform gauze

5. Positioning:

    Supine with arm extended out on arm board and hand prone

6. Technique:

    a. Sterile prep and drape finger and hand.
    b. Digital block per section II B. If severe inflammation, digital block may be ineffective and patient may require injections surrounding paronychia..
    c. If paronychial fold and only small part of adjacent eponychium involved:
       • Elevate only the lateral 1/3 nail closest to side of infection from nail bed with fine Halsted clamp or fine scissors (see Figure 8.12).
       • Cut nail longitudinally with fine scissors to isolate 1/3 of nail to be removed, as shown in diagram.
       • Free up 1/3 of eponychium from nail by spreading fine Halsted clamp or fine scissors under eponychium.
       • Remove this separated nail.
    d. If infection is more extensive, remove entire nail per section III A.
    e. Incise eponychial fold to promote drainage if necessary.
    f. Irrigate wound with saline using a 30-ml syringe and 19-gauge angiographic catheter, and soak wound in dilute Betadine for 5 minutes prior to dressing wound.
    g. Dress wound with Xeroform to keep nail bed covered and skin edges open.

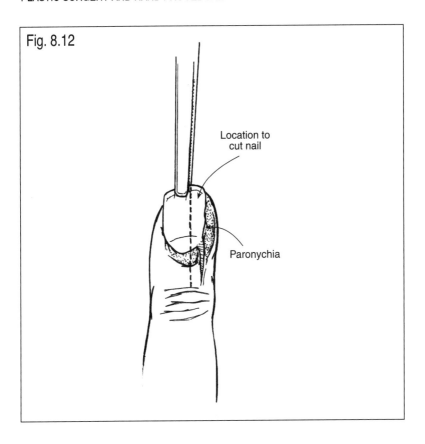

Fig. 8.12

Location to cut nail

Paronychia

h. Continue saline soaks for 15 minutes twice daily until healed.

7. Complications and Management:
   a. Inadequate drainage
      • Incise eponychial fold.
      • If still inadequate, remove nail per section III A.
   b. Nail bed injury: Repair per section III B.

E. INCISION AND DRAINAGE OF UPPER EXTREMITY ABSCESS

1. Indications:

   Superficial hand/forearm abscesses

2. Contraindications:

a. Suspected deep abscesses may require radiologic guidance of ultrasound versus computed tomography to evaluate or drain.

b. Abscess near important neurovascular structures.

3. Anesthesia:

Local/field block

4. Equipment:

a. Sterile prep solution
b. Sterile gloves and towels
c. Scalpel
d. Halsted clamp
e. Sterile saline
f. Gauze
g. Syringe
h. 25-gauge and 18-gauge needles
i. Cast padding
j. Plaster or fiberglass for splint

5. Positioning:

Supine with arm extended out on arm board

6. Technique:

a. Sterile prep and drape hand or forearm.
b. Administer anesthesia.
c. Aspirate over area of greatest fluctuance with 18-gauge needle to localize abscess and obtain a sample for microbiology if deemed necessary.
d. Make an adequate incision over area of greatest fluctuance with scalpel. May need to make narrow elliptical incision to promote drainage.
e. Break up loculations with a Halsted clamp. Define borders of abscess if possible (see Figure 8.13).
f. Irrigate copiously with saline using saline bottle as a squirt bottle. Punch holes in the top with 18-gauge needle. Pack the cavity with gauze or iodoform strip gauze.
g. Splint the forearm/hand in the position of function. See Chapter 9, Orthopedic Procedures.

Fig. 8.13

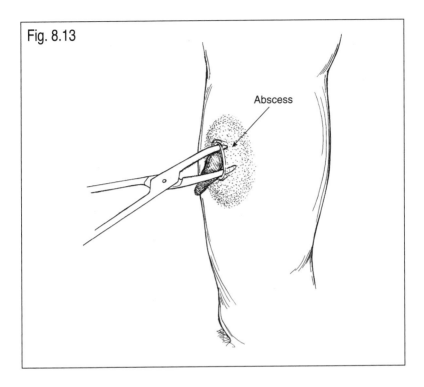

Abscess

7. Complications and Management:
   a. Inadequate drainage
      • Deep abscesses may require radiologic guided or operative drainage.
   b. Neurovascular injury
      • Observe.
      • May need operative repair.

F. HAND FRACTURES, SUBLUXATIONS, AND DISLOCATIONS

All fractures should be referred to a hand specialist for follow-up.

1. Indications:
   a. Radiographically documented subluxation (incomplete joint separation) or dislocation (complete joint separation) of the phalanges at the distal interphalangeal joint (DIP), proximal

interphalangeal joint (PIP), or metacarpophalangeal (MCP) joints, without demonstrable joint instability.

b. Radiographically documented fracture of the distal tuft; distal, middle, or proximal phalangeal shaft; metacarpal head, neck, shaft or base; and thumb metacarpal fractures, both intra-articular and extra-articular.

2. Contraindications:

Splint and refer the following to a hand surgeon.

a. Open dislocation or fracture
b. Intra-articular fracture or oblique fracture of condylar heads of a phalanx
c. Fracture subluxations
d. Multiple hand fractures
e. Joints with demonstrable instability should be immobilized in a radial or ulnar gutter splint (see Chapter 9).

3. Anesthesia:

Digital block if DIP/PIP joint or distal/middle/proximal phalanx (see section I B), wrist block if MCP or metacarpal (see section I C)

4. Equipment:

Appropriate splint for immobilization of affected part (see below)

5. Positioning:

Supine with arm extended on arm board, palm down

6. Technique:

a. Perform thorough physical examination, checking vascular, neurological, and flexor and extensor tendon integrity.
b. Determine position of subluxation or dislocation by physical examination and radiologic assessment, either lateral, dorsal, or volar (based on distal segment position); stress roentgenograms may be helpful.
c. After anesthesia is administered, perform systematic evaluation of joint stability actively and passively, with radial and ulnar stress to each collateral ligament and posterior—anterior stress to volar plate in extended and moderately flexed positions.

d. Fractures
- Distal phalanx fractures: Assess for nail bed and extensor
  tendon injury.
  (1) Tuft—Commonly associated with soft tissue injury to
      the nail bed. Reduce tuft fracture and repair nail bed as
      described in section III B. Fracture immobilization is
      rarely necessary, but a small splint excluding the PIP
      joint (see Figure 8.14) is frequently used for 2–3 days to
      protect the distal phalanx from further trauma.

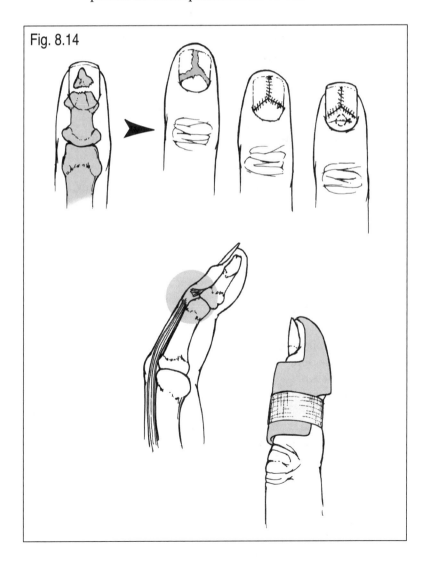

Fig. 8.14

(2) Shaft—Closed reduction with dorsal traction, if necessary, and splint with volar stack or frog splint (see Figure 8.14). Irreducible fractures should be referred to a hand surgeon for K-wire fixation.

(3) Base—Can be associated with flexor or extensor tendon avulsion.

- Proximal and middle phalangeal fractures: Assess for any malrotation or scissoring (see Figure 8.15). Stable, nondisplaced fractures can be buddy-taped (see Figure 8.15) to allow for early protected motion within the first 3–5 days. If there is any displacement or instability (common with oblique fractures), attempt closed reduction with dorsal traction. These fractures require precise, anatomic alignment because of the relationship with the extensor and flexor tendons. For injuries of the little or ring finger, immobilize in the position of function in an ulnar gutter splint. For injuries of the long and index fingers, immobilize in the position of function in a volar or radial gutter splint (see Chapter 9).

e. Subluxations and dislocations

- Distal interphalangeal joint: Relatively uncommon location for dislocations, but may be associated with an open wound. If an open wound is present, irrigate thoroughly and repair wound after reduction. If dislocated, position is usually dorsal. Digital block is necessary before closed reduction. Apply longitudinal traction and hyperextend distal segment followed by direct dorsal pressure to the base of the distal phalanx. Assess for stability with active and passive range of motion. Immobilize the DIP joint only in a stack or short volar splint (see Figure 8.14). If an open wound is present, splint in slight DIP joint flexion with a dorsal splint for 3 weeks. Consider prophylactic antibiotics.
- Proximal interphalangeal joint: Most commonly dorsal or lateral (ulnarly deviated) position. Assess for concomitant avulsion fractures. Digitally block involved digit. Closed reduction of a dorsal dislocation is easily accomplished by longitudinal traction with hyperextension to disengage the middle phalanx. Apply direct pressure to the proximal volar aspect of the middle phalanx (see Figure 8.16). Lateral dislocations are reduced with longitudinal traction, mild accentuation of the displaced segment (either ulnarly or radially), and direct pressure on the proximal aspect of

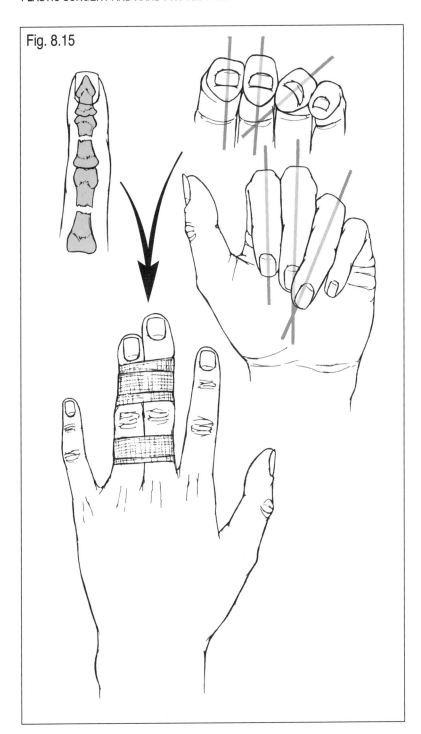

Fig. 8.15

Fig. 8.16

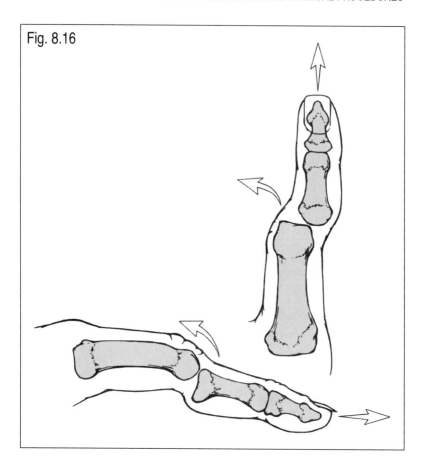

the middle phalanx directed toward desired position of phalanx. Volar dislocations are generally irreducible by closed reduction and require the expertise of a hand surgeon. Assess for stability with active and passive range of motion. Immobilize in 30° of flexion with a volar or frog-leg splint.

- Interphalangeal joint of the thumb (IP): Similar to DIP dislocation (see above). Usually in the dorsal position. Apply median nerve block to anesthetize and reduce as described in the DIP section above. After reduction, assess for stability with active and passive range of motion, and immobilize in mild flexion with a volar splint (see Chapter 9).

IV. COMPLEX LACERATIONS

A. LIP

1. Indications:

   Lip laceration

2. Contraindications:

   Laceration greater than 1/3 of lip length

3. Anesthesia:

   Local/field block/facial block (see section I D)

4. Equipment:

   a. Sterile prep solution
   b. Sterile gloves and towels
   c. 25-gauge needle
   d. 5-ml syringe
   e. Sterile saline
   f. Scalpel
   g. 4-0 chromic suture
   h. 4-0 Vicryl suture
   i. 6-0 nylon suture
   j. Laceration tray—fine scissors, clamp, tissue forceps, needle driver

5. Positioning:

   Supine

6. Technique:

   a. Sterile prep and drape lip and lower face.
   b. Administer local anesthesia.
   c. Trim edges of wound with scalpel or scissors if necessary and copiously irrigate wound with saline.
   d. If laceration is full-thickness, it must be closed in three layers (see Figure 8.17).
      • Muscle: Approximate with one or two simple interrupted 4-0 vicryl sutures.

Fig. 8.17

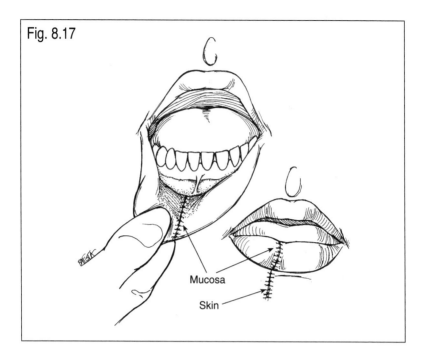

Mucosa

Skin

- Skin: Approximate edges with simple interrupted 6-0 nylon sutures, carefully aligning the skin-vermilion border.
- Mucosa: Approximate with simple interrupted 4-0 chromic sutures.

B. EAR

1. Indications:

Simple ear laceration

2. Contraindications:

a. Grossly contaminated or human bite wounds should not be immediately closed.

b. Amputated or near amputated ears require operative repair.

3. Anesthesia:

Local/field block/auricular block (see section I E)

4. Equipment:

a. Sterile prep solution
b. Sterile gloves and towels
c. 25-gauge needle
d. Syringe
e. Laceration tray—fine scissors, clamp, tissue forceps, needle driver
f. Scalpel
g. 5-0 nylon suture
h. 4-0 Dexon suture
i. Xeroform gauze
j. 4 × 4-inch gauze, fluffed gauze, 3-inch Kling gauze
k. 3-inch Ace wrap

5. Positioning:

Supine with head turned to one side

6. Technique:

a. Sterile prep and drape ear.
b. If the laceration involves skin and only a small cartilage defect, skin approximation is all that is needed to restore the auricular contour.
   - Approximate the skin with simple interrupted 5-0 nylon sutures.
   - If the laceration involves the rim of the ear, use a vertical mattress suture with 5-0 nylon along the rim to evert the edges, which will prevent a notched appearance at the rim (see Figure 8.18).
c. If there is a larger cartilage defect, first close the cartilage with simple interrupted 4-0 Dexon suture and tie the knots on the posterior side.
d. If a hematoma is present below the skin of the external ear, drain the hematoma by making a small incision with the scalpel over the hematoma.
e. Apply a compressive ear dressing:
   - Pack Xeroform strips into ear crevices.
   - Tuck a 4 × 4-inch gauze behind the ear.
   - Place a wad of fluffed gauze over the ear.
   - Wrap head and injured ear with a 3-inch Kling followed by a 3-inch Ace wrap, leaving the opposite ear free of dressing.

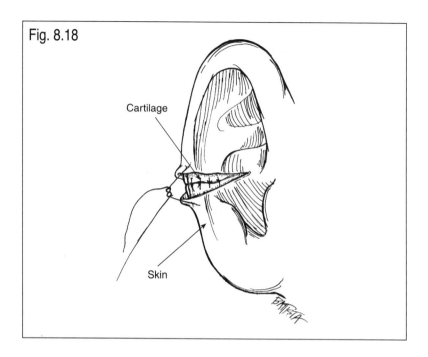

Fig. 8.18

Cartilage

Skin

7. Complications and Management:
   a. Hematoma
      Check wound in 24 hours. If a hematoma develops, it must
      be drained and a compressive dressing reapplied.
   b. Later complications include chondritis, stricture of external
      auditory canal, and keloid formation.

V. DERMABOND TOPICAL SKIN ADHESIVE

A. DERMABOND, 2-OCTYL CYANOACRYLATE, IS A STERILE, LIQUID TOPICAL ADHESIVE.

1. Indications:
   a. Superficial lacerations with no irregular shape
   b. Can be used after placement of subcutaneous dermal sutures

2. Contraindications:
   a. Stellate or irregular-shaped wounds

b. Lacerations on hair-bearing skin
c. Contaminated wounds or wounds resulting from a bite
d. Mucosal or mucosal junction wounds
e. Wounds usually closed with 4-0 nylon or larger suture

3. Anesthesia:

Local/field if necessary

4. Equipment:

a. Sterile prep solution
b. Sterile gloves
c. Dermabond

5. Technique:

Clean the skin with antiseptic and irrigate as if closing the wound with suture. Before application, clean the surface with alcohol and let dry. Approximate wound edges closely with fingers and forceps. Break the sterile applicator containing the bonding material. Apply an initial coat with a 10–30 second delay, then reapply multiple layers covering 5–10 mm outside the wound edges. Mean time to drying is approximately 1 minute. No external bandage or antibiotic ointment is necessary. Polymer begins to peel off 7 days after application.

6. Complications:

a. Infection
b. Dehiscence of wound

CHAPTER 9

ORTHOPEDIC PROCEDURES

Author: Chandrakanth Are, M.D.

ORTHOPEDIC PROCEDURES

This chapter describes the management of some of the commonly encountered orthopedic injuries. Acknowledging that there is more than one method of handling each injury, some of the commonly used methods are outlined.

I. MEASUREMENT OF COMPARTMENT PRESSURES

1. Indications:
   a. Any condition that increases pressure within an osteofascial compartment and causes neurovascular compromise, such as hematoma due to fractures, muscle swelling due to ischemia, etc.
   b. More commonly seen in the leg and forearm, rarely in the thigh.
   c. Common clinical signs:
      • Pain with passive motion of the muscles (early sign)
      • Increasing pain and pain out of proportion to injury
      • Pallor
      • Paresthesia
      • Paralysis (late sign)
      • Pulselessness (lack of pulse is a late and unreliable sign)

2. Contraindications:
   a. Coagulopathy
   b. Infection at puncture site

3. Anesthesia:

  a. None.
  b. Injection of local anesthetic can increase intracompartmental pressures.
  c. Intravenous (IV) sedation prevents monitoring of clinical situation.

4. Equipment:

  a. Stryker pressure and monitoring kit
  b. Whiteside's technique:
  - Sterile 20-ml Luer lock syringe
  - Four-way stopcock
  - Bottle of sterile saline
  - 35-Inch extension tubes (two)
  - 18-Gauge needles (two)
  - Mercury thermometer

5. Positioning:

Extremity to be measured is horizontal to ground and resting on flat surface

6. Technique—Whiteside's Technique for Calf Pressures:

  a. Assemble apparatus as shown, with a 20-ml syringe (see Figure 9.1).
  b. Insert needle into the bottle of sterile saline with stopcock closed to manometer.
  c. Aspirate saline until half of the extension tube is filled.
  d. Sterile prep and drape calf.
  e. Insert 18-gauge needle into the muscle of compartment to be measured.
  - Anterior compartment: muscle mass just lateral to the ridge of tibia
  - Lateral compartment: just anterior to the fibula
  - Superficial posterior compartment: From medial aspect of calf, enter posterior muscle belly approximately 2–5 cm in depth, depending on patient's subcutaneous fat
  - Deep posterior compartment: From position of superficial posterior compartment, angle anteriorly and advance needle into deep tissue
  f. Open stopcock to both extension tubes and syringe.

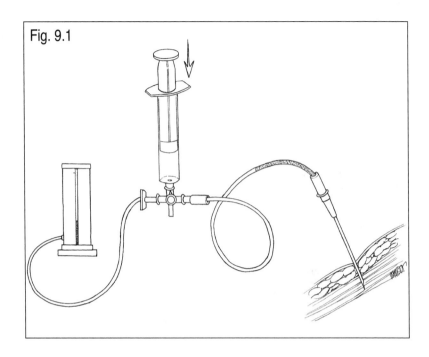

Fig. 9.1

g. Slowly depress syringe plunger until air/saline meniscus moves.
h. When air/saline meniscus moves, read pressure in manometer and record.
i. Withdraw needle and enter next compartment to be measured.
j. When in doubt as to accuracy of readings, the uninjured contralateral extremity can be used as a control.
k. Technique can be modified to any compartment of the body.
l. Place sterile gauge over the puncture site.
m. If pressure is greater than 40 mm Hg, fasciotomy is indicated.

7. Complications:
   a. Error in reading—double check each reading
      • Ensure manometer and extremity are level.
      • Compare to opposite extremity.
      • If borderline, remeasure pressure 1–2 hours later.
   b. Infection—local wound care and antibiotics

II. ARTHROCENTESIS, INTRA-ARTICULAR AND PERIARTICULAR INJECTIONS

1. Indications:
   a. Diagnostic
      • Septic arthritis
      • To differentiate inflammatory and noninflammatory conditions such as trauma and osteoarthritis
      • To diagnose crystalloid arthritis
      • Synovial biopsy
   b. Therapeutic
      • For intra-articular injection
      • To aspirate large effusions
      • For lavage of joints

2. Contraindications:
   a. Local infection such as overlying cellulitis.
   b. Systemic infection with possible bacteremia (aspiration may be performed under the cover of antibiotics if deemed urgent).
   c. Coagulopathy, hemophilia.
   d. Allergy to substance injected.
   e. Aspiration of prosthetic joint is better left to be done by the surgeon under strict aseptic conditions.
   f. Joints with severe distortion that are unlikely to respond are a relative contraindication.

3. Anesthesia:
   1% lidocaine subcutaneously

4. Equipment:
   a. Sterile prep set
   b. Sterile gloves and drapes
   c. 18-gauge needle for large joints
   d. 25-gauge needle for small joints
   e. 20-ml syringes (two)
   f. 5-ml syringes for injection
   g. Small Kelly clamp
   h. One EDTA (lavender top) and one heparinized (green top) sample tube

     i. Culture swabs

    j. 1% Lidocaine

5. Positioning:

   a. Metacarpophalangeal joints: Rest pronated hand on table and flex joint by 45°.

   b. Wrist joint: Rest pronated wrist on table.

   c. Carpal tunnel syndrome: Rest supinated hand on table.

   d. Elbow joint: Rest elbow on table in flexed position with forearm pronated.

   e. Shoulder joint: Patient should be sitting with the arm hanging by the side and the elbow flexed 90°.

   f. Knee and ankle joints: Rest knee or ankle in stretcher.

6. Approaches:

   a. Metacarpophalangeal joints: Inject on dorsal surface. Feel for the transverse groove on either of the extensor tendons along the joint line. Enter the joint in this groove with a 25-gauge needle. Appropriate injection is confirmed by ballooning of the joint (see Figure 9.2).

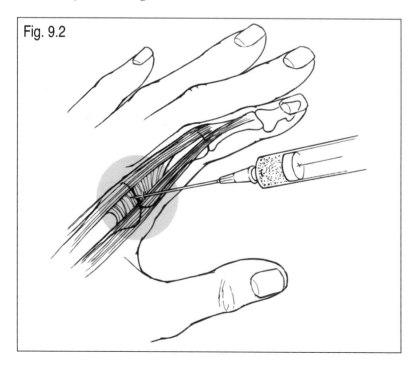

Fig. 9.2

b. Wrist joint: Insert needle at the base of snuff box just adjacent to the radial aspect of extensor pollicis longus. The snuff box can be palpated with the thumb in extension (see Figure 9.3).

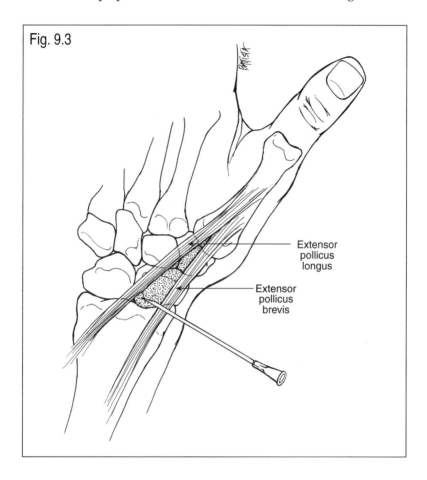

Fig. 9.3

Extensor
pollicus
longus

Extensor
pollicus
brevis

c. Carpal tunnel syndrome: Inject on volar surface. Palmarflex the hand against resistance to make the tendons of palmaris longus and flexor carpii radialis prominent. The palmaris longus lies on the ulnar side of the latter. Inject between these tendons just proximal to the distal crease with the needle pointing distally. If the patient feels a sharp severe electrical pain, the needle tip is in the nerve; withdraw the needle. Do not inject the nerve. Correct injection is confirmed by anesthesia in the area of distribution of the median nerve (see Figure 9.4).

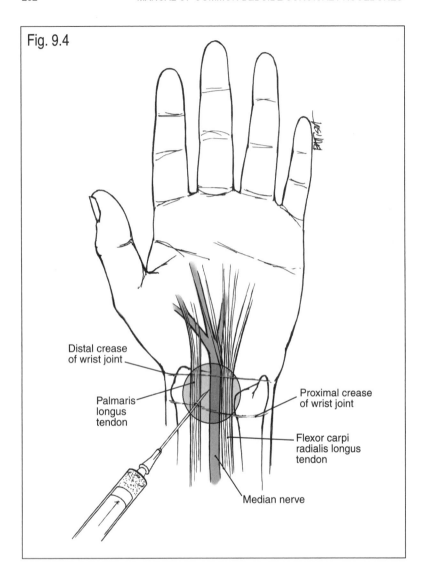

Fig. 9.4

Distal crease of wrist joint

Palmaris longus tendon

Proximal crease of wrist joint

Flexor carpi radialis longus tendon

Median nerve

d. Elbow joint: Insert needle at posterior aspect just lateral to the olecranon (see Figure 9.5).

e. Shoulder joint: Mark a triangle with the coracoid process as the medial point, tubercle of the head of the humerus as the lateral point, and tip of the acromion as the superior point. Insert the needle at the center of the triangle to a depth of 1–2 cm with the needle pointing posteriorly. May need to rotate

Fig. 9.5

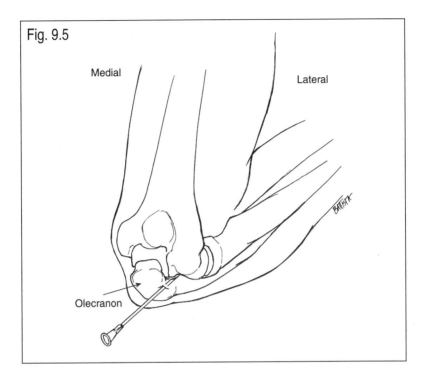

Medial

Lateral

Olecranon

arm internally and externally to find entrance point (see Figure 9.6).

f. Knee joint: Insert needle laterally at level of superior pole of patella, then advance into the joint (see Figure 9.7).

g. Ankle joint: Insert needle 2.5 cm proximal and 1.3 cm medial to the tip of the lateral malleolus (see Figure 9.8).

7. Technique:

a. Place patient in comfortable position, preferably supine.

b. Optimal joint position is important for stretching the capsule and the articular surfaces apart.

c. Identify landmarks and ascertain the point of needle entry.

d. Clean skin with povidone iodine and prep the entire joint.

e. Inject 1% lidocaine subcutaneously at point of needle entry and raise a wheal with a 25-gauge needle.

f. With a longer needle, inject lidocaine into the periarticular tissues.

g. Spraying the skin with cold ethylchloride may also provide adequate anesthesia.

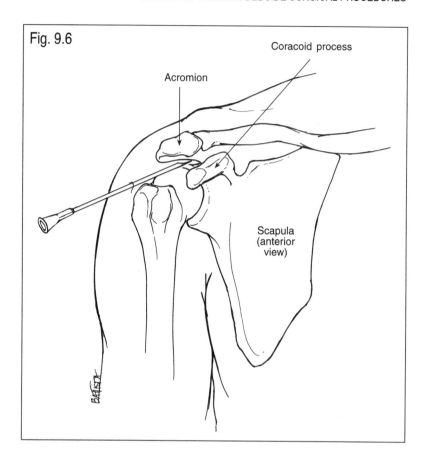

Fig. 9.6

Coracoid process

Acromion

Scapula
(anterior
view)

h. Attach 18-gauge needle to a large syringe and insert into the joint.
i. Aspirate, and if syringe is full, stabilize needle with a Kelly clamp to enable exchange of syringe.
j. Flow of fluid can be interrupted at times due to clogging by synovium or debris. Rotating the needle, withdrawing it slightly, or even re-injecting some fluid can help declog.
k. If joint injection is to be done, it should be done only after complete aspiration. Correct injection into joint is confirmed by feeling little or no resistance to injection.
l. Send fluid for evaluation:
   • Lavender tube: cell count and differential
   • Green tube: crystal analysis
   • Culture swabs: Gram stain and C/S

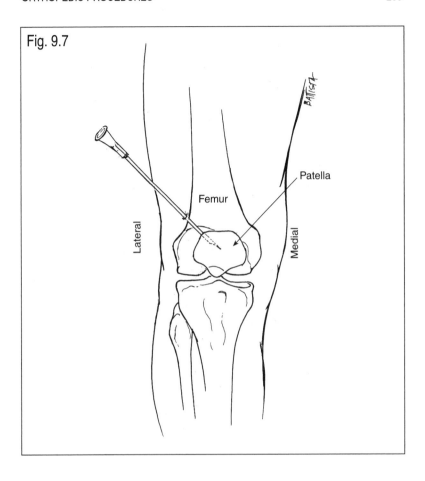

Fig. 9.7

m. Advise rest of affected joint for 2–3 days, especially the weight-bearing joints.

8. Complications:
   a. Infection: Treat with antibiotics.
   b. Intra-articular and periarticular bleeding: Treat with pressure dressing and rest.
   c. Allergic reaction: Treat as for anaphylaxis.
   d. Postinjection flare (symptoms worsen temporarily after injection): Treat with rest, ice, and nonsteroidal anti-inflammatory drugs.
   e. Cutaneous atrophy (due to lipolytic action of steroids): Skin appearance will return to normal as the steroid is completely absorbed.

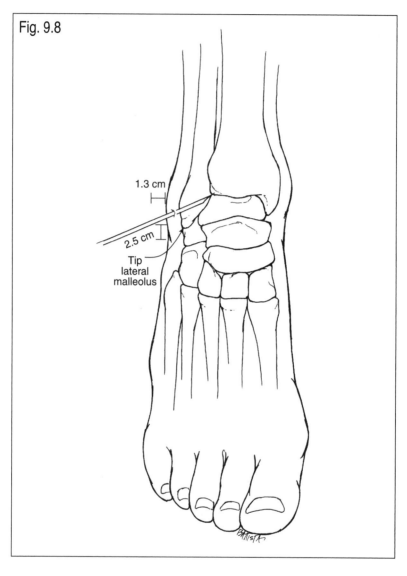

Fig. 9.8

1.3 cm

2.5 cm

Tip
lateral
malleolus

f. Tendon rupture is due to repeated injections into the tendon, which should be avoided.

g. Weakness of extremity due to injection of the nerve will resolve spontaneously.

h. Vasovagal syncope may occur.

i. Steroid arthropathy: Avoid repeat injections.

j. Avascular necrosis: Avoid repeat injections.

k. Steroid-induced osteoporosis: Avoid repeat injections.

9. Dosage and Administration:

a. Steroids available:
- Hydrocortisone: usual range, 25–100 mg
- Prednisolone tebutate: usual range, 5–40 mg
- Methylprednisolone acetate: usual range, 4–40 mg
- Triamcinolone acetonide: usual range, 5–40 mg

Prednisone is the least expensive, and triamcinolone derivatives are the least water soluble with least systemic absorption and longest duration of action.

b. Rough guide for doses (prednisone):
- Small joints of hand and foot: 2.5–10 mg
- Medium joints (elbow and wrist): 10–25 mg
- Knee, ankle, shoulder: 20–50 mg
- Hip: 30–50 mg

Interval between injections should be at least 4 weeks.

III. SPLINTING

1. Indications:

a. Fracture
b. Dislocated joint after reduction
c. Sprain: torn or stretched ligaments
d. Strain: torn or stretched muscles or tendons
e. Postoperative immobilization

2. Contraindications:

a. Absolute: none.
b. Relative: Injuries involving open wounds or infections need easily removable splints to allow soft tissue care.

3. Anesthesia:

If injury is grossly stable, use IV sedation (see Appendix C).

4. Equipment:

a. Cast padding (soft roll)
b. Plaster/fiberglass
c. Lukewarm water
d. Ace bandages
e. Disposable gloves

5. Positioning:

   a. Ankle/foot: 90° angle between foot and leg, neutral eversion/inversion
   b. Knee: 15°–20° flexion
   c. Shoulder: resting at the side of the body
   d. Elbow: 90° angle between forearm and arm, neutral pronation/supination
   e. Wrist: neutral supination/pronation, 20°–30° wrist extension
   f. Thumb: wrist position as above, thumb in 45° abduction, 30° flexion
   g. Metacarpals, MCP joint, proximal phalanges: wrist position as above, MCP joint in 90° flexion, DIP and PIP joints in full extension
   h. IP joints, middle/distal phalanx: full extension at IP joints

6. Technique:

   a. Splint padding
   - Apply cast padding to entire area to be splinted with 2–3 inches of proximal and distal overhang.
   - Padding should be applied evenly in a circular fashion from distal to proximal, with each turn overlapping by 50% of the next turn to allow at least two layers of padding in all areas (see Figure 9.9).
   - Apply extra layers to bony prominences.
   - Apply padding while limb is in final splint position to prevent bunching of padding across joint flexion creases.
   b. Fiberglass/plaster
   - General technique: Immobilize fracture one joint above and one joint below injury.
   - Prefabricated fiberglass splints can be measured and cut.
   - Plaster splints need 10–12 layers of plaster in upper extremities and 12–15 layers of plaster in lower extremities.
   - Splints are dipped in room-temperature or lukewarm water.
   - Excess water is gently squeezed or shaken from the splint.
   - Splint is applied to the soft roll and never directly onto the skin. The splint is held in place by an assistant or the patient.
   c. Ace wrap
   - Wrap Ace bandage around splint with gentle tension.
   - Ace wrap should never be tight enough to cause venous compression.
   - Hold extremity in desired position until splint hardens

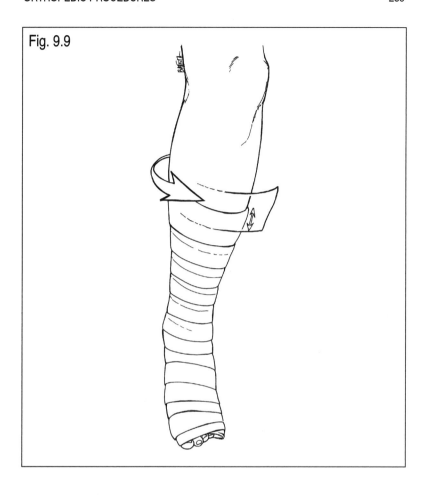

Fig. 9.9

(approximately 5–10 minutes with fiberglass, 10–15 minutes with plaster).

7. Specific Splints:

a. Posterior elbow splint (see Figure 9.10)
   - Begin 4-inch-wide splint from posterior upper arm, moving across the posterior elbow.
   - Extend the splint over the ulnar border of the forearm and hand to just proximal to the MCP joint.

b. Sugar tong forearm splint (see Figure 9.11)
   - Use for forearm / wrist injuries.
   - Begin with 3- to 4-inch-wide splint in the palm of the hand at the level of the MCP joints.

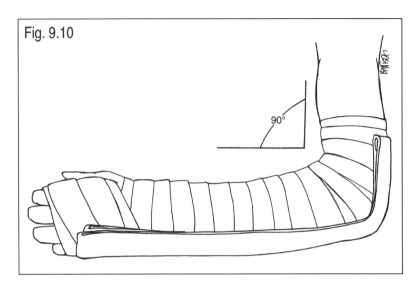

Fig. 9.10

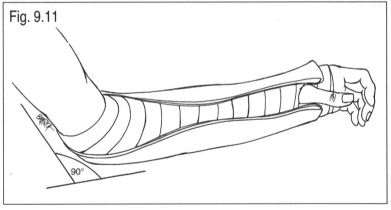

Fig. 9.11

- Extend splint up dorsal aspect of the forearm, around the elbow flexed at 90°, down the volar aspect of the forearm and hand, to just proximal to the MCP joint.
- Be sure that the splint does not limit MCP motion.
  c. Ulnar gutter splint (see Figure 9.12)
    - Used for fourth and fifth metacarpal or phalanx injuries.
    - Apply 3- to 4-inch-wide slab from ulnar aspect of proximal forearm down along the ulnar aspect of the small finger.
    - Fold edges around dorsal and volar aspect of hand and ring/small fingers.
    - Place the wrist in neutral supination/pronation with 20°–30° extension.

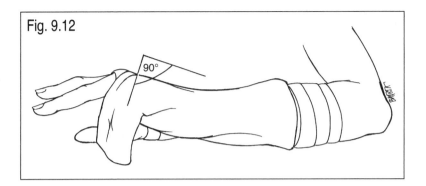

Fig. 9.12

d. Radial gutter splint (see Figure 9.13)
  • Used for injuries of the second/third metacarpal or fingers.
  • Apply to radial border as above for ulnar side with a hole cut out to allow motion of the thumb.
  • Alternatively, apply two separate 2- to 3-inch-wide slabs to volar and dorsal aspect of hand and fingers.

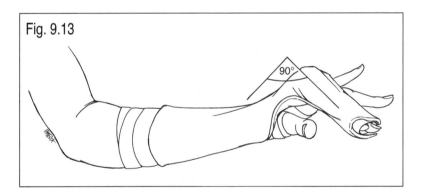

Fig. 9.13

e. Thumb spica splint (see Figure 9.14)
  • Apply sugar tong splint as above.
  • Add an additional 3-inch-wide slab from upper forearm, along radial border, then down around thumb.
  • Thumb IP joint should be included.
f. Long leg splint (see Figure 9.15)
  • Used for knee and tibia injuries.
  • Apply 4-inch-wide splint beginning at the medial upper thigh and extending down the medial knee and ankle.
  • Continue the splint around the heel and up the lateral side

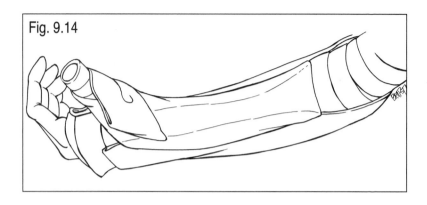

Fig. 9.14

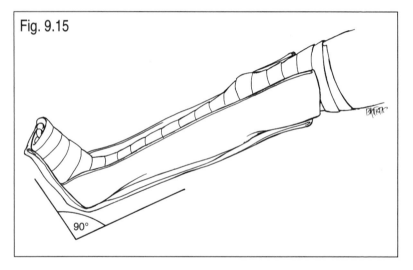

Fig. 9.15

90°

of the ankle and knee to the lateral upper thigh, forming a
U shape.
- For additional stability, apply a 6-inch splint from the
posterior upper thigh down to the posterior aspect of the
leg and plantar surface of the foot.
g. Ankle splint (see Figure 9.16)
- Use for isolated ankle injuries.
- Apply 4-inch-wide splint beginning at the proximal border
of the upper calf, extending down the medial calf and
ankle, and around the heel and up the lateral ankle and
lateral calf.
- For additional stability, apply a 6-inch splint from the
posterior upper calf down the posterior aspect of the lower
leg and the plantar surface of the foot.

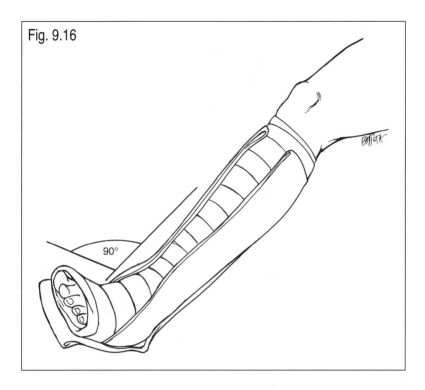

Fig. 9.16

8. Complications and Management:

  a. Burns
- Splints harden by exothermic reaction and can burn underlying skin.
- Be sure skin is properly padded.
- Never use hot water to moisten splints.
- Avoid overly thick splints.
- If patient complains of significant heat or pain, remove splint and check the underlying skin.
- If burn occurs, treat with local burn techniques including debridement and topical Silvadene as necessary.

  b. Cast sores
- Compression of skin over extended periods can lead to necrosis and breakdown.
- Be sure all bony and tendinous prominences are well padded.
- Be cautious about applying splints in unconscious patients or patients with insensate skin.
- If patient complains of burning pain or discomfort, remove splint and inspect skin.

- If splint is foul-smelling or drainage appears, remove splint immediately and inspect.
- If wound develops, treat with local wound care.
- Avoid indenting the splint with finger pressure while it is hardening.

c. Joint contracture
  - Long-term immobilization can lead to shortening of ligaments and tendons if improperly positioned.
  - Check and re-check position of splint as it hardens.
  - Avoid immobilization for longer than 3 weeks for shoulder and elbow injuries; 6 to 8 weeks for any other injury.
  - If contracture develops, begin physical therapy immediately.
  - Orthopedics consult.

IV. CLOSED JOINT REDUCTION

Always assess neurovascular status before and after reduction. Always obtain a radiograph of the entire involved bone to rule out an associated fracture that may be detrimental to the reduction, for example, the entire humerus in shoulder dislocation, etc.

A. SHOULDER JOINT DISLOCATION

This is one of the most commonly encountered injuries.

1. Indications:
   a. Anterior dislocation
   b. Posterior dislocation

2. Contraindications:
   a. Associated fracture of the humeral shaft
   b. Associated fracture of the greater tuberosity in itself is not a contraindication to the initial treatment, although it may merit subsequent attention.

3. Anesthesia:
   IV sedation (see Appendix C)

4. Equipment:
   Shoulder immobilizer

5. Positioning:
   a. Anterior dislocation—Matson's method: Patient lies supine with head of the bed elevated by 30° with the injured side close to the edge of the bed.
   b. Anterior dislocation—Stimson's method: Patient lies prone at the edge of the table with a sandbag under the clavicle.
   c. Posterior dislocation—Same as for Matson's method.

6. Technique:
   a. Anterior dislocation—Matson's method (see Figure 9.17)
      • Assess neurovascular status with particular attention to the axillary nerve.
      • A sheet folded into a 5-inch swath is wrapped around the

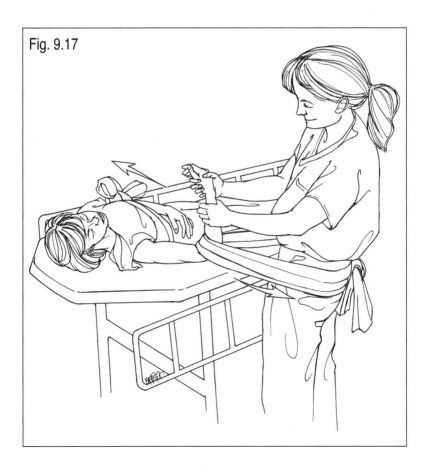

Fig. 9.17

patient's thorax and tied to the bed rails to provide countertraction, or held by an assistant if available.

- A second sheet is loosely wrapped around the surgeon's waist.
- The physician stands on the injured side and passes the forearm into the second sheet, holding the forearm in 90° flexion at the elbow and 25°–30° abduction at the shoulder joint.
- Traction and countertraction are applied in the line of the arm with the physician leaning on the sheet around the waist.
- Sustained traction is applied over a period of several minutes, which should reduce the dislocation with a click.
- To this basic maneuver is added gentle rocking of the humerus from internal to external rotation.
- Reduction can also be helped by adding outward pressure on the head of the humerus from the axilla.
- Confirm reduction clinically by the following: The prominence of the deltoid muscle returns, the head of the humerus can no longer be felt below the coracoid process, and the patient will be able to touch the opposite shoulder with the hand of the injured side.
- Immobilize the shoulder in internal rotation and adduction in an immobilizer, with the aim of avoiding abduction and external rotation.
- Confirm reduction by x-ray in both AP and Y views.
- The duration of immobilization is 2–5 weeks for younger people, and less for patients older than 40 years to avoid stiffness.

b. Stimson's method

- This method may be applied when adequacy of personnel may be an issue.
- The arm hangs free off the table with appropriate weights attached at the wrist.
- Ten pounds is usually sufficient, but more weight may be required for heavier patients.
- It usually takes 20–30 minutes to achieve reduction, and reduction is considered failed if there is no result in 1 hour.
- It is important not to leave the patient unattended, particularly after administration of sedation.

c. Posterior dislocation

- These injuries are rare and more difficult to reduce than anterior dislocations.

- They can be reduced by the same traction–countertraction method as described above.
- Axial traction is applied in the line of the arm.
- Gentle internal rotation will unlock the humeral head from the glenoid rim and facilitate reduction.
- Lateral traction on the proximal humerus will also help unlock the humeral head.
- Once unlocked, gentle external rotation will achieve reduction.
- Avoid forcible external rotation, which can cause humeral fracture.
- Reduction is confirmed clinically and by x-ray.

7. Complications and Management:
   a. Fractures
   b. Unable to reduce dislocation
   c. Injury to axillary nerve
      - Splint as needed
      - Orthopedics consult

B. RADIAL HEAD DISLOCATION

This injury is more common in children. Isolated dislocation of the radial head in adults is very rare and is usually a part of Monteggia fracture dislocation.

1. Indications:
   Isolated dislocation or subluxation of the radial head

2. Contraindications:
   Associated fracture of the radial shaft

3. Anesthesia:
   IV sedation (see Appendix C)

4. Equipment:
   Sling

5. Positioning:
   Patient can be either sitting or lying down.

6. Technique:

Technique is illustrated in Figure 9.18.

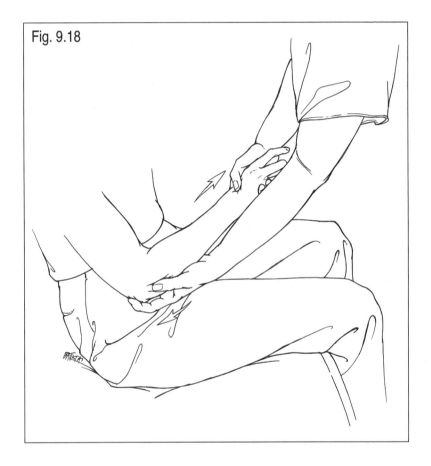

Fig. 9.18

a. The physician holds the patient's injured hand in a hand-shake position.
b. Place the other hand behind the elbow with the thumb on the radial head to apply pressure in the posterior direction.
c. While applying traction on the arm combined with pressure on the radial head, supinate the forearm to achieve reduction.
d. If this fails, alternatively pronate and supinate the forearm to help reduction.
e. Rest the arm in a sling afterward.

7. Complications and Management:

Unable to reduce—orthopedic consult

C. HIP DISLOCATIONS

Hip dislocation implies a significant force of injury; therefore, care should be taken to rule out other associated injuries.

1. Indications:

Posterior dislocation

2. Contraindications:

a. Associated fracture of the femoral neck
b. Associated fracture of the femoral shaft

3. Anesthesia:

IV sedation (see Appendix C)

4. Equipment:

Skin traction kit

5. Positioning:

Supine

6. Technique:

Technique is illustrated in Figure 9.19.
a. Always assess neurovascular status with particular attention to the sciatic nerve.
b. Patient lies supine.
c. An assistant stands on the side opposite the injury and steadies the pelvis by applying pressure on the anterior superior iliac spine in the posterior direction.
d. The affected limb is gently flexed to 90° at the knee and hip at the same time.
e. While performing the above maneuver, the internal rotation and adduction deformity that accompanies posterior dislocation is corrected.

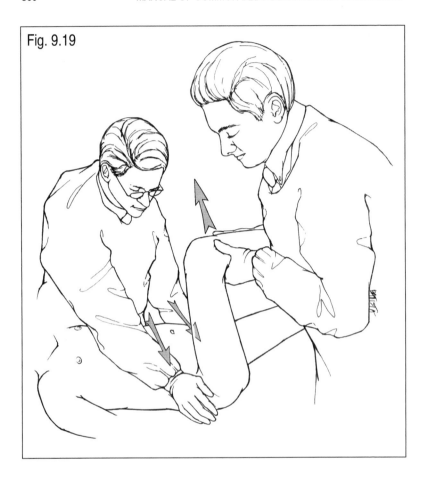

Fig. 9.19

f. In this position, traction is applied in the line of the femur while the pelvis is kept steady, which may require the physician to stand on the table.

g. Reduction is achieved with a clunk and is confirmed by radiology.

h. After reduction, the limb is placed in skin traction.

7. Complications:
   a. Injury to sciatic nerve
   b. Irreducible dislocations
   c. Fracture of femoral neck

D. ANKLE DISLOCATION

Always obtain radiographs of the entire tibia and fibula. Reduction should be achieved emergently to avoid compromise to neurovascular structures and the skin. This may sometimes have to be done without any sedation or analgesia to avoid delays.

1. Indications:

Clinically or radiographically dislocated joint

2. Contraindications:

Tibial shaft fracture

3. Anesthesia:

IV sedation (see Appendix B)

4. Equipment:

a. Cast padding (soft roll)
b. Plaster/fiberglass
c. Lukewarm water
d. Ace bandages
e. Disposable gloves

5. Positioning:

Patient lying on stretcher with legs hanging over the end to let gravity assist in the reduction.

6. Technique:

Technique is illustrated in Figure 9.20.

a. Have an assistant stabilize the legs by placing his/her hands on the patient's thighs.
b. Grasp the forefoot with one hand and the heel with the other hand.
c. Recreate the mechanism of injury by twisting the foot toward the side to which the talus is dislocated.
d. Reverse the mechanism of injury to pull the talus back under the tibia.

Fig. 9.20

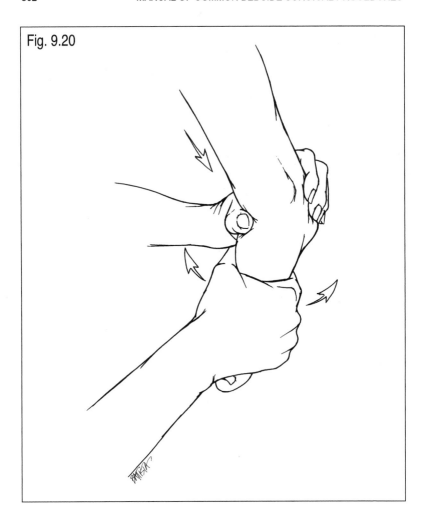

7. Complications and Management:

Unable to reduce—orthopedic consult.

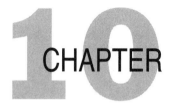

CHAPTER

NEEDLE BIOPSIES

Authors: Andrew L. Singer, M.D., and Attila Nakeeb, M.D.

NEEDLE BIOPSIES

Needle biopsy is a powerful technique that is most often used to distinguish malignant from benign disease. Recently it has given the clinician the ability to follow the progression of many benign processes, such as transplant rejection. With ready access to ultrasound, the surgeon can now safely sample both palpable and nonpalpable lesions at the bedside or in the outpatient office.

Needle biopsy can be divided into two general categories: (1) fine needle aspiration (FNA), in which a fine needle is inserted into the tissue and a collection of single cells is obtained for cytological diagnosis, and (2) large needle cutting biopsies (LNCB), in which a large cutting needle retrieves a cylinder of tissue for histological diagnosis. The major shortcoming of both techniques is that when small samples are obtained they may inadequately represent the tissue being sampled. However, in skilled hands, needle biopsy is a sensitive, inexpensive, and relatively noninvasive modality for the evaluation of pathology of the head and neck, thyroid, breast, liver, kidney, pancreas, and subcutaneous and muscular masses.

I. FINE NEEDLE ASPIRATION

A. THYROID

1. Indications:
   a. Evaluation of palpable thyroid masses
   b. Differentiation of benign from malignant thyroid lesions

2. Contraindications:

None

3. Anesthesia:

Anesthesia is not routinely used for FNA. However, if needed, a small amount of 1% lidocaine may be infiltrated locally, taking care not to distort the palpable lesion.

4. Equipment:

   a. Alcohol prep
   b. 10-ml syringe
   c. 1/2-inch 25-gauge needle
   d. Syringe holder (optional)
   e. Glass microscope slides (two)
   f. Spray fixative, gauze
   g. In many situations, it may be preferable to have a cytopathologist present.

5. Positioning:

The patient is placed in a supine position, and a roll is placed behind the shoulders to allow for neck extension and to bring the lesion closer to the surface (see Figure 10.1).

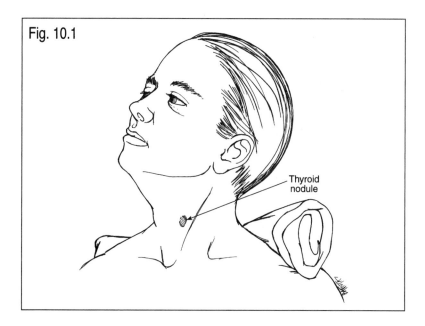

Fig. 10.1

Thyroid nodule

6. Technique:

a. Prep the area for aspiration with an alcohol prep pad as if for phlebotomy.

b. Palpate the lesion and immobilize the mass between the fingertips of the nondominant hand (see Figure 10.2).

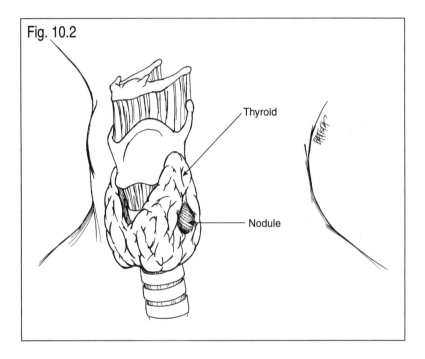

Fig. 10.2

Thyroid

Nodule

c. Using the dominant hand, advance a 25-gauge needle with an attached 10-ml syringe into the lesion. The needle should be directed medially, toward the trachea (see Figure 10.3).

d. Note the consistency of the mass upon entering it with the needle (firm, soft, rubbery, doughy, gritty).

e. Once the lesion is entered, a full 10 ml of suction is applied to the syringe. In a variant of this procedure, the nonsuction technique, no negative pressure is applied to decrease local trauma and bleeding.

f. While maintaining suction (if used), move the needle back and forth through the lesion several times in different directions (see Figure 10.4).

g. Release the syringe plunger and allow it to return to a neutral position prior to removing the needle from the lesion. In the nonsuction technique, the plunger will already be in neu-

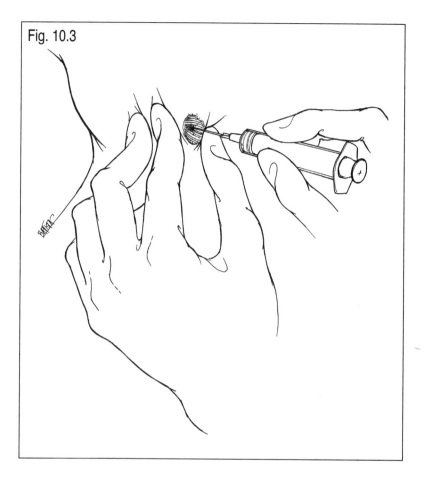

Fig. 10.3

tral position. At this point the specimen is within the needle
and hub and should not be in the syringe.

h. Remove the needle from the patient, and have the patient
apply pressure to the puncture site with a gauze pad.

i. Detach the needle from the syringe.

j. Fill the syringe with air.

k. Reattach the needle onto the syringe.

l. Touch the needle tip to a glass microscope slide with the
bevel at a 45°–90° angle to the slide surface.

m. Expel material within the needle onto the slide.

n. Make a smear by using a second glass slide to gently press
down and draw out the material to a feathered edge. If the
material is more liquid, it is pulled in the same fashion as a
blood smear, except that before the feathering process is
completed, the spreading slide is raised, leaving a line of

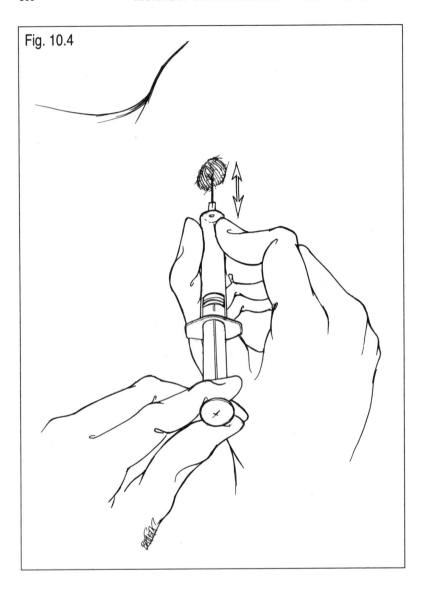

Fig. 10.4

particles across the slide. The spreading slide is then turned
and again pressed down against the line of particles and
drawn out into a feathered edge.
o. Air dry or apply cytological fixative to the slide per the protocol of the cytopathology laboratory that will be processing
the specimen. (If a fixative is applied, it must be applied very
quickly, usually within seconds of preparing the smear.)

p. Most cytopathologists require 3–6 needle passes (samples) for an adequate pathological diagnosis.

q. If a cyst is aspirated, the cyst fluid should be sent for cytology. The region of the cyst should then be re-examined; if a residual mass is felt, it should then undergo FNA.

7. Complications and Management:

a. Bleeding and hematomas
   - Thyroid punctures may produce significant hematomas and ecchymoses.
   - Apply firm direct pressure to puncture sites immediately following aspiration.

b. Tracheal puncture
   - If the trachea is entered, the suction in the syringe will be lost, and the aspiration will need to be repeated.
   - Puncture is usually of no consequence due to the small gauge of the needle.

c. Infection
   - Extremely rare in FNA but has been reported
   - Antibiotics as appropriate
   - Incision and drainage as necessary

B. BREAST, LYMPH NODE, AND SOFT TISSUE

1. Indications:

a. Evaluation of palpable masses
b. Aspiration of breast cysts
c. Differentiation of benign from malignant lesions. In breast disease, stereotactic large-gauge needle biopsy by radiologists has become the technique of choice for evaluation of breast lesions. However, FNA continues to be a valid technique and is essential for centers lacking stereotactic facilities.

2. Contraindications:

None

3. Anesthesia:

Anesthesia is not routinely used for FNA. However, if needed, a small amount of 1% lidocaine may be infiltrated locally, taking care not to distort the palpable lesion.

4. Equipment:
   a. Alcohol prep
   b. 10-ml syringe
   c. 1 1/2-inch 25-gauge needle
   d. Syringe holder (optional)
   e. Glass microscope slides (two)
   f. Spray fixative
   g. Gauze

5. Positioning:
   a. Breast: For upper quadrant lesions, the patient is placed in an upright seated position. Lower quadrant lesions are better managed in a supine position.
   b. Lymph node and soft tissue: depends on location of lesion.

6. Technique:
   a. Prep the area for aspiration with an alcohol prep pad as if for phlebotomy.
   b. Palpate the lesion and immobilize the mass between the fingertips of the nondominant hand.
   c. Using the dominant hand, advance a 25-gauge needle with an attached 10-ml syringe into the lesion (see Figure 10.5).

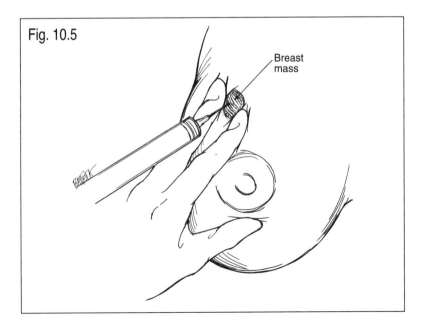

Fig. 10.5

Breast mass

d. Note the consistency of the mass upon entering it with the needle (firm, soft, rubbery, doughy, gritty).
e. Once the lesion is entered, a full 10 ml of suction is applied to the syringe.
f. While maintaining suction, move the needle back and forth through the lesion several times in different directions (see Figure 10.6).
g. Release the syringe plunger and allow it to return to a neutral position prior to removing the needle from the lesion. At

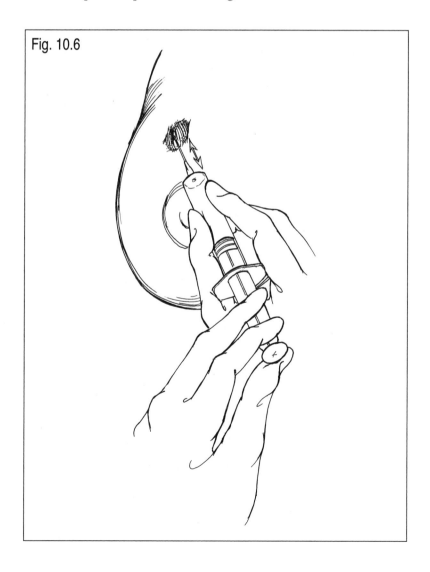

Fig. 10.6

this point the specimen is within the needle and hub and should not be in the syringe.

h. Remove the needle from the patient, and have the patient apply pressure to the puncture site with a gauze pad.

i. Detach the needle from the syringe.

j. Fill the syringe with air.

k. Reattach the needle onto the syringe.

l. Touch the needle tip to a glass microscope slide with the bevel at a 45°–90° angle to the slide surface.

m. Expel material within the needle onto the slide.

n. Make a smear by using a second glass slide to gently press down and draw out the material to a feathered edge. If the material is more liquid, it is pulled in the same fashion as a blood smear, except that before the feathering process is completed, the spreading slide is raised, leaving a line of particles across the slide. The spreading slide is then turned and again pressed down against the line of particles and drawn out into a feathered edge.

o. Air dry or apply cytological fixative to the slide per the protocol of the cytopathology laboratory that will be processing the specimen. (If a fixative is applied, it must be applied very quickly, usually within seconds of preparing the smear.)

p. Most cytopathologists require 3–6 needle passes (samples) for an adequate pathological diagnosis.

q. If a cyst is aspirated, the cyst fluid should be sent for cytology. The region of the cyst should then be re-examined; if a residual mass is felt, it should then undergo FNA.

7. Complications and Management:

a. Bleeding and hematomas
   - Breast FNA can be associated with significant hematomas and ecchymoses.
   - Apply firm direct pressure to puncture sites immediately following aspiration.

b. Pneumothorax
   - More likely in thin patients and deep lesions
   - If tension pneumothorax suspected, decompression with 16-gauge intravenous line (IV) into second intercostal space and then tube thoracostomy (see Chapter 4)
   - If 10% to 20% pneumothorax, observation and serial chest radiographs
   - If >20% pneumothorax, tube thoracostomy per Chapter 4

c. Infection
- Extremely rare in FNA but has been reported
- Antibiotics as appropriate
- Incision and drainage as necessary

II. LARGE NEEDLE CUTTING BIOPSIES

A. SILVERMAN NEEDLE BIOPSY (SOFT TISSUE)

1. Indications:
To differentiate benign and malignant lesions

2. Contraindications:
Coagulopathy (PT or PTT ratio >1.3 times control, or platelets <20,000)

3. Anesthesia:
1% lidocaine locally

4. Equipment:
a. Sterile prep solution
b. Sterile gloves and towels
c. 5-ml syringe
d. 22- and 25-gauge needles
e. Scalpel blade
f. Silverman needle (see Figure 10.7)
g. Sterile dressing

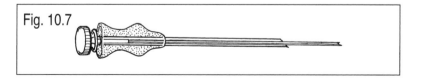

Fig. 10.7

5. Positioning:
The best patient position is when the lesion can be easily palpated and fixed into place by the examiner using one hand. For most biopsies the supine position is preferred. In thyroid and neck

aspirations a roll is placed behind the shoulders, which allows for neck extension and brings the lesion closer to the surface.

6. Technique:

   a. Sterile prep and drape the lesion to be biopsied.
   b. Infiltrate the skin overlying the lesion with 1% lidocaine, using a 25-gauge needle.
   c. Using the 22-gauge needle, infiltrate the subcutaneous tissue down to the mass with anesthetic.
   d. Make a 5-mm incision in the skin and subcutaneous tissue with a scalpel.
   e. Insert the Silverman needle with the obturator in place into the skin incision to the edge of the mass.
   f. Remove the obturator, and place the cutting insert into the outer sheath and advance into the mass (see Figure 10.8).

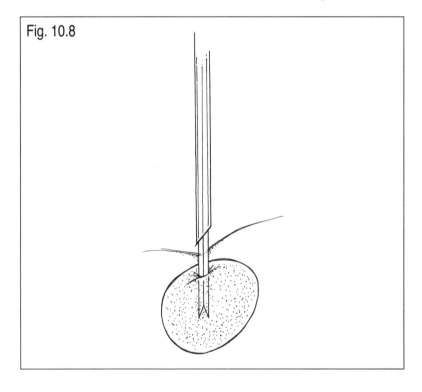

Fig. 10.8

   g. Advance the outer sheath by rotation over the cutting insert to the tip. This maneuver severs the specimen within the blades of the cutting insert (see Figure 10.9).

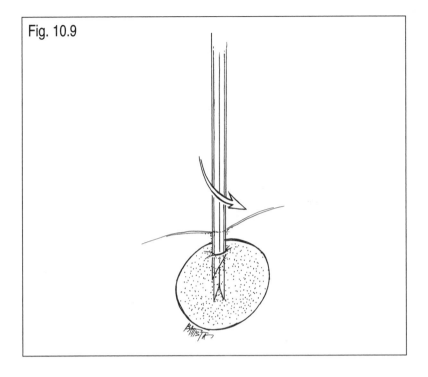

Fig. 10.9

h. Remove the needle with the outer sheath advanced over the cutting insert. Retrieve the specimen and send to pathology for processing.
i. Apply a clean sterile dressing to wound and apply pressure for 20–30 minutes.

7. Complications and Management:
   a. Bleeding and hematomas
      • Apply firm direct pressure to puncture sites immediately following aspiration.
      • Correct coagulation abnormalities.
   b. Infection
      • Antibiotics as appropriate
      • Incision and drainage as necessary

B. TRU-CUT NEEDLE BIOPSY (SOFT TISSUE)

1. Indications:

   To differentiate benign and malignant lesions

2. Contraindications:

Coagulopathy (PT or PTT ratio >1.3 times control, or platelets <20,000)

3. Anesthesia:

1% lidocaine locally

4. Equipment:

   a. Sterile prep solution
   b. Sterile gloves and towels
   c. 5-ml syringe
   d. 22- and 25-gauge needles
   e. Scalpel blade
   f. Tru-cut needle (see Figure 10.10)

Fig. 10.10

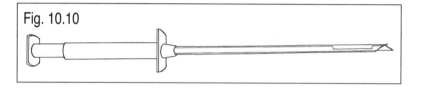

   g. Sterile dressings

5. Positioning:

The best patient position is when the lesion can be easily palpated and fixed into place by the examiner using one hand. For most biopsies the supine position is preferred. In thyroid and neck aspirations a roll is placed behind the shoulders, which allows for neck extension and brings the lesion closer to the surface.

6. Technique:

   a. Sterile prep and drape the lesion to be biopsied.
   b. Infiltrate the skin overlying the lesion with 1% lidocaine using a 25-gauge needle.
   c. Using the 22-gauge needle, infiltrate the subcutaneous tissue down to the mass with anesthetic.
   d. Make a 5-mm incision in the skin and subcutaneous tissue with a scalpel.
   e. Fully retract the obturator of the Tru-cut needle so that the specimen notch is covered (see Figure 10.11).

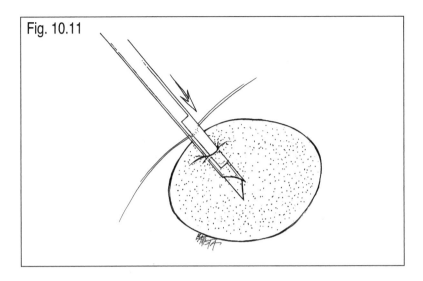

Fig. 10.11

f. Insert the needle into the lesion so that the specimen notch is within the lesion to be biopsied (see Figure 10.12).

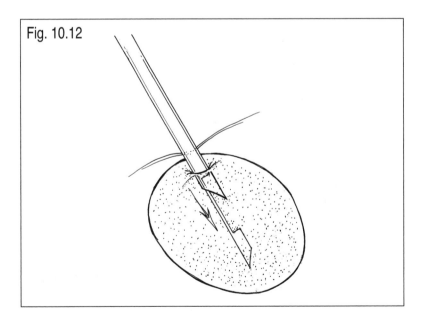

Fig. 10.12

g. Hold the obturator in place and pull outward on the T-shaped cannula handle to expose the specimen notch.

h. Quickly but carefully advance the T-shaped cannula handle over the obturator to sever the tissue that has prolapsed into the open specimen notch (see Figure 10.13).

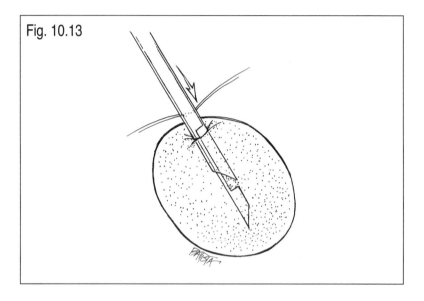

Fig. 10.13

i. Remove the Tru-cut needle with the cannula in the advanced position over the obturator.
j. Advance the obturator to expose the specimen notch and re-move the tissue for pathology.
k. Apply a clean sterile dressing to wound and apply pressure for 20–30 minutes.

7. Complications and Management:
   a. Bleeding and hematomas
      • Apply firm direct pressure to puncture sites immediately following aspiration.
      • Correct coagulation abnormalities.
   b. Infection
      • Antibiotics as appropriate
      • Incision and drainage as necessary

C. PERCUTANEOUS LIVER BIOPSY

1. Indications:
   a. Diagnosis of primary liver disease
   b. Assessment of the progression of chronic liver disease
   c. Detection of malignant primary or metastatic disease
   d. Documentation of rejection in liver transplant patients

2. Contraindications:
   a. Uncooperative patient
   b. Coagulopathy (PT or PTT ratio >1.3 times control, or platelets <30,000)
   c. Local infection
   d. Massive tense ascites

3. Anesthesia:
   1% lidocaine locally

4. Equipment:
   a. Sterile prep solution
   b. Sterile gloves and towels
   c. 5-ml syringe
   d. 22- and 25-gauge needles
   e. Scalpel blade
   f. Tru-cut biopsy needle
   g. Sterile dressing

5. Positioning:
   Percutaneous liver biopsy is performed with the patient in the supine position with the patient's right arm tucked behind the head. Warn the patient of the possibility of sharp pain with radiation to the right shoulder.

6. Technique:
   a. Map the liver by percussion (or ultrasound). Mark the biopsy site on the skin 2–3 cm above the caudal margin of the liver in the midaxillary line (see Figure 10.14).

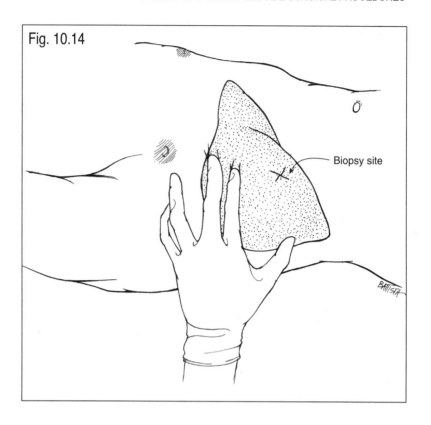

Fig. 10.14

Biopsy site

b. Sterile prep and drape the right upper quadrant of the abdomen.
c. Infiltrate the skin with 1% lidocaine over the biopsy site.
d. Using a 22-gauge needle, infiltrate the subcutaneous tissue with local anesthetic. With a scalpel blade, make a 5-mm skin incision.
e. Fully retract the obturator of the Tru-cut needle so that the specimen notch is covered.
f. Ask the patient to take a deep breath and hold it.
g. Insert the needle into the liver so that the specimen notch is within the lesion to be biopsied. The needle should only need to be inserted 2–4 cm.
h. Ask the patient to exhale and hold his or her breath.
i. Hold the obturator in place and pull outward on the T-shaped cannula handle to expose the specimen notch.
j. Quickly but carefully advance the T-shaped cannula handle over the obturator to sever the tissue that has prolapsed into the open specimen notch.

    k. Remove the Tru-cut needle with the cannula in the advanced position over the obturator.

    l. Advance the obturator to expose the specimen notch and remove the tissue for pathology.

    m. Apply a clean sterile dressing to wound and apply pressure for 20–30 minutes.

    n. Patient should lie on the right side for at least 2 hours.

7. Complications and Management:

    a. Bleeding and hematoma
- Apply firm direct pressure to puncture sites immediately following aspiration.
- Correct coagulation abnormalities.
- Surgical exploration if necessary.

    b. Infection
- Antibiotics as appropriate
- Incision and drainage as necessary
- Operative drainage as necessary

    c. Pneumothorax
- More likely in thin patients and deep lesions
- If tension pneumothorax suspected, decompression with 16-gauge IV into second intercostal space and then tube thoracostomy (see Chapter 4)
- If 10%–20% pneumothorax, observation and serial chest radiographs
- If >20% pneumothorax, tube thoracostomy per Chapter 4

D. PERCUTANEOUS KIDNEY BIOPSY

1. Indications:

    a. Diagnosis of primary renal disease

    b. Assessment of the progression of chronic renal disease

    c. Documentation of rejection in renal transplant patients

2. Contraindications:

    a. Uncooperative patient

    b. Coagulopathy (PT or PTT ratio >1.3 times control, or platelets <30,000)

    c. Severe uncontrolled hypertension

    d. Known or suspected renal parenchymal infection

e. Solitary ectopic or horseshoe kidney (except renal transplant)

3. Anesthesia:

1% lidocaine locally

4. Equipment:

a. Sterile prep solution
b. Sterile gloves and towels
c. 5-ml syringe
d. 22- and 25-gauge needles
e. Scalpel blade
f. Biopsy needle (Silverman or Tru-cut needle)
g. Sterile dressing
h. Ultrasound
i. Locating needle (22-gauge spinal needle)

5. Positioning:

Percutaneous renal biopsy is performed with the patient in the prone position with a roll placed under the patient between the rib cage and the pelvis. Transplant biopsies are performed with the patient in a supine position.

6. Technique:

a. Sterile prep and drape the appropriate flank area.
b. Confirm the position of the kidney by ultrasound. Using a 25-gauge needle, infiltrate the skin with 1% lidocaine over the biopsy site (lower pole of kidney).
c. Using a 22-gauge needle, infiltrate the subcutaneous tissue with local anesthetic.
d. Make a 5-mm incision through the skin and subcutaneous tissue with a scalpel blade.
e. Ask the patient to hold his or her breath in inspiration, and advance the locating needle under ultrasound guidance into the kidney.
f. Release the needle and ask the patient to breathe in and out normally. If the needle is in proper position, the end of the needle will move in a cephalad direction on inspiration and in a caudal direction on expiration.

g. Determine the depth of the kidney by measuring the distance from the needle tip to where it exits the skin.
h. Remove the locating needle, and advance the Silverman or Tru-cut needle into the kidney at the same angle and depth as the locating needle using the techniques described in sections II A or II B.

7. Complications and Management:

a. Bleeding and hematomas
 • Apply firm direct pressure to puncture sites immediately following aspiration.
 • Correct coagulation abnormalities.
b. Infection
 • Antibiotics as appropriate
 • Incision and drainage as necessary
 • Operative drainage as necessary
c. Pneumothorax
 • More likely in thin patients and deep lesions
 • If tension pneumothorax suspected, decompression with 16-gauge IV into second intercostal space and then tube thoracostomy (see Chapter 4)
 • If 10%–20% pneumothorax, observation and serial chest radiographs
 • If >20% pneumothorax, tube thoracostomy per Chapter 4

E. PERCUTANEOUS PANCREAS BIOPSY

1. Indications:

Diagnosis of rejection and allograft viability in transplant patients in whom the pancreas has been anastomosed with urinary drainage

2. Contraindications:

a. Uncooperative patient
b. Coagulopathy (PT or PTT ratio >1.3 times control, or platelets <30,000)
c. Severe pancreatitis in transplanted organ
d. Enterically drained pancreas allograft. Although these organs can be percutaneously biopsied, it is traditionally done in the ultrasound suite by radiologists and not at bedside by surgeons.

3. Anesthesia:

   1% lidocaine locally

4. Equipment:

   a. Sterile prep solution
   b. Sterile gloves and towels
   c. 5-ml syringe
   d. 22- and 25-gauge needles
   e. Scalpel blade
   f. Biopsy needle (Silverman or Tru-cut needle)
   g. Sterile dressing
   h. Ultrasound
   i. Locating needle (22-gauge spinal needle)

5. Positioning:

   Supine

6. Technique:

   a. Sterile prep and drape the abdomen.
   b. Confirm the position of the pancreas allograft by ultrasound (see Figure 10.15). Using a 25-gauge needle, infiltrate the skin over the biopsy site with 1% lidocaine.
   c. Using a 22-gauge needle, infiltrate the subcutaneous tissue with local anesthetic.
   d. Make a 5-mm incision through the skin and subcutaneous tissue with a scalpel blade.
   e. Ask the patient to hold his or her breath in inspiration, and advance the locating needle under ultrasound guidance into the pancreas allograft.
   f. Release the needle and ask the patient to breathe in and out normally.
   g. Determine the depth of the pancreas by measuring the distance from the needle tip to where it exits the skin.
   h. Remove the locating needle, and advance the Silverman or Tru-cut needle into the allograft at the same angle and depth as the locating needle using the techniques described in sections II A or II B.

7. Complications and Management:

   a. Bleeding and hematomas
      • Apply firm direct pressure to puncture sites immediately following aspiration.

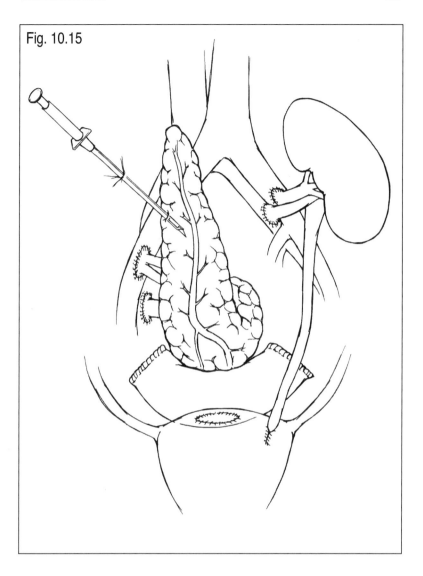

Fig. 10.15

- Correct coagulation abnormalities.
- Given the density of vascular structures in the area of the allograft, operative repair can be necessary in the event of inadvertent large vessel laceration.

b. Infection
- Antibiotics as appropriate
- Incision and drainage as necessary
- Operative drainage as necessary

APPENDIX A
LIFE SUPPORT PROTOCOLS

Author: Glen S. Roseborough, M.D.

Resuscitation protocols for treating life-threatening cardiac and trauma emergencies have been developed by the American Heart Association and the American College of Surgeons. Physicians and other health care professionals are trained to follow these protocols in courses offered by the two institutions at regular intervals and at various locations in North America and around the world, as other countries have adopted these protocols as the standard of care. These courses, Advanced Cardiac Life Support (ACLS) and Advanced Trauma Life Support (ATLS), provide the trainee with a basic framework through which he or she can assess and treat a patient suffering from a cardiac emergency or multisystem trauma, and do so in an efficient, systematic manner. Course participants receive instruction in all the relevant diagnostic and therapeutic procedures that are covered elsewhere in this book, with priority given to management of the airway, pulmonary and cardiovascular systems is stressed. Recertification in ACLS and ATLS is recommended every 3 to 4 years. In the following pages the basic protocols taught in these courses are summarized.

ADVANCED CARDIAC LIFE SUPPORT

All physicians will encounter cardiac arrhythmias during their careers, so familiarity with ACLS protocols for management of these problems is essential. Rapid diagnosis and institution of treatment is critical because the probability of successfully treating a malignant arrhythmia decreases rapidly with time; of patients presenting with witnessed collapse and ventricular fibrillation as their initial rhythm, survival decreases from 30% with early cardiopulmonary resuscitation (CPR) and defibrillation to only 2%–8% when defibrillation is delayed up to 10 minutes. The treating physician must be familiar with the techniques of CPR, defibrillation with the automatic external defibrillator, cardiac pacing, intubation, and obtaining intravenous access. One must also be able to recognize the life-threatening arrhythmias, including ventricular tachycardia, ventricular fibrillation, pulseless electrical activity, asystole, bradycardia, and supraventricular tachycardia, as well as know how to use the medications to treat these arrhythmias. More recently protocols have been added that address management of acute myocardial infarction and pulmonary edema; these will be omitted in this appendix.

ACLS (and ATLS) algorithms begin by evaluating the patient with a primary and secondary survey. In the primary survey, the rescuer focuses on basic CPR and defibrillation; in the secondary survey, one performs a more detailed assessment and carries out additional therapeutic interventions. The order of these interventions is prioritized by following the ABCs of resuscitation (airway, breathing, circulation): control of the airway, ensuring ventilation and oxygenation with 100% oxygen, and maintaining perfusion with volume expansion and vasoactive/cardioactive drugs. When intravenous access is unobtainable, the following drugs may be administered via an endotracheal tube: naloxone, atropine, diazepam (Valium), epinephrine, and lidocaine (remember as NAVEL).

The protocols for treating the basic arrhythmias are represented in the flowsheets presented in Figures 1–4. They can be summarized as follows. Asystole and pulseless electrical activity are treated with epinephrine and atropine. Ventricular fibrillation and ventricular tachycardia are treated with defibrillation/unsynchronized cardioversion, epinephrine, and lidocaine. Bretylium, magnesium sulfate, and procainamide may be given additionally if the patient does not respond to epinephrine and lidocaine. Bradyarrhythmias are treated with pacing and chromotropes (atropine, dopamine, isoproterenol, or epinephrine). Supraventricular (i.e., narrow complex) tachycardias are treated with synchronized cardioversion if unstable, then adenosine followed by a calcium channel blocker, beta blocker, digoxin, or procainamide. CPR should be initiated and maintained throughout the resuscitation if the patient is found to be pulseless or profoundly hypotensive, and the patient should be rechecked for the return of pulses after each intervention.

In most instances the resuscitation may be terminated if no vital signs are established within 30 minutes of its beginning; the chances of survival beyond this point are minimal. Exceptions to this rule may include children and patients subjected to hypothermia, electrocution, and drug overdose.

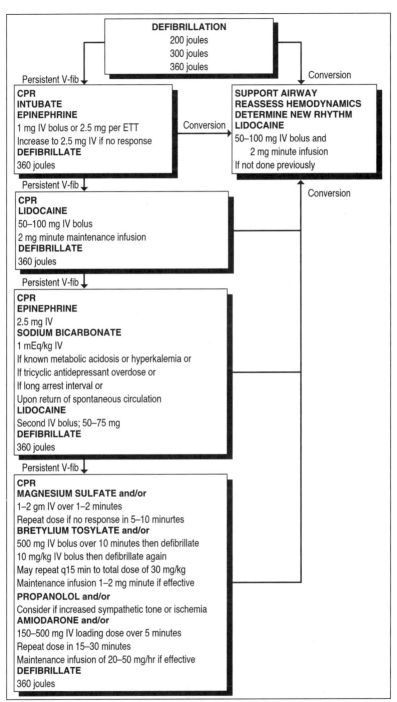

FIGURE 1. Algorithm for treatment of adult ventricular fibrillation. Modified from Grauer K, Cavallaro D. An approach to the key algorithms for cardiopulmonary resuscitation. In: Welmer RA, Scardiglia J, eds. ACLS Certification Preparation. St. Louis: Mosby Lifeline, 1993:3–38.

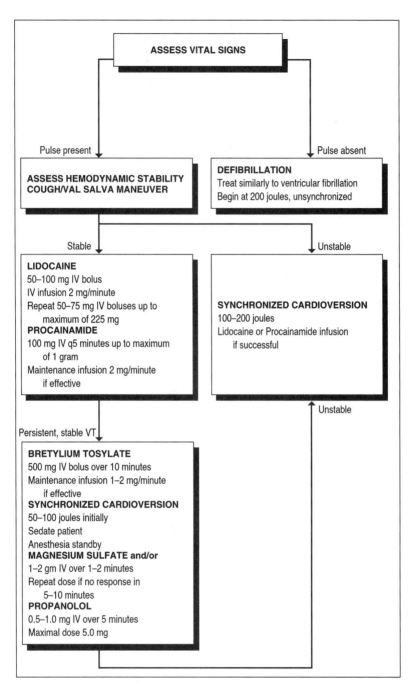

FIGURE 2. Algorithm for treatment of adult sustained ventricular tachycardia. Modified from Grauer K, Cavallaro D. An approach to the key algorithms for cardiopulmonary resuscitation. In: Welmer RA, Scardiglia J, eds. ACLS Certification Preparation. St. Louis: Mosby Lifeline, 1993:3–38.

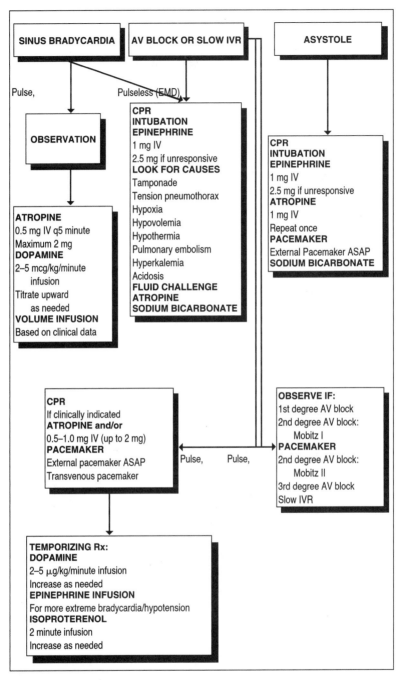

FIGURE 3. Algorithm for treatment of adult bradycardia, EMD, and asystole. Modifed from Grauer K, Cavallaro D. An approach to the key algorithms for cardiopulmonary resuscitation. In: Welmer RA, Scardiglia J, eds. ACLS Certification Preparation. St. Louis: Mosby Lifeline, 1993:3–38.

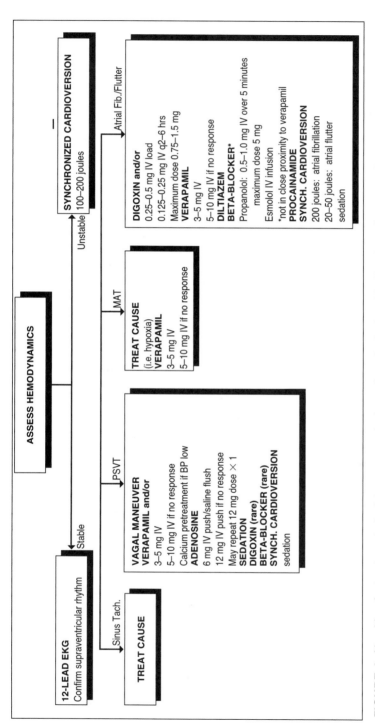

FIGURE 4. Algorithm for treatment of adult supraventricular tachyarrhythmias. Modified from Grauer K, Cavallaro D. An approach to the key algorithms for cardiopulmonary resuscitation. In: Welmer RA, Scardiglia J, eds. ACLS Certification Preparation. St. Louis: Mosby Lifeline, 1993:3–38. *Legend: PSVT,* paroxysmal supraventricular tachycardia; *MAT,* multifocal atrial tachycardia.

ADVANCED TRAUMA LIFE SUPPORT

Trauma accounts for the leading cause of death between the ages of 1 and 44 years, and is the third leading cause of death overall. This amounts to about 150,000 deaths annually in the United States, and more than three times that number of people become permanently disabled as a result of trauma. The overall cost of caring for trauma patients exceeds $400 billion annually.

Caring for the multiply injured trauma patient is a daunting task for the untrained physician. The timing of death from trauma occurs in a trimoidal distribution: (1) within seconds to minutes of injury, death results from major injury to the brain, brain stem, spinal cord, heart, aorta, or other major blood vessels; (2) within minutes to hours of injury, death results from subdural or epidural hematomas, cardiac tamponade, hemopneumothorax, spleen or liver lacerations, pelvic fractures, and various injuries associated with significant blood loss; (3) within days to weeks of injury, death is usually caused by sepsis and multiple organ dysfunction syndrome. ATLS focuses on maximizing patient care and survival in the second set of patients, during the "golden hour" or first hour after injury occurs. Treatment starts by evaluating the patient with a primary and secondary survey. During the primary survey, life-threatening conditions are identified and management is instituted simultaneously in order of priority determined by what will kill the patient the fastest. This order is reflected in the "ABCDE" of resuscitation:

A. Airway and cervical spine protection
B. Breathing (ventilation and oxygenation)
C. Circulation—control external bleeding, obtain intravenous access
D. Disability (neurological status)
E. Exposure (undress patient) and environment (temperature control)

A secondary survey is then performed, consisting of a head-to-toe examination of the patient, at which time one can document and address more site-specific injuries. Adjunctive investigations such as radiographs, blood work, and urine samples are obtained at this point, and urinary catheters and nasogastric tubes are placed if necessary. From this point on, the patient should be continuously monitored (vital signs, electrocardiogram, oxygen saturation, urine output, etc.), and the response to each intervention should be observed. It is critical to

continuously re-evaluate the patient who is not responding as
expected to a given intervention (i.e., a fluid bolus or placement
of a chest tube) to avoid missing an occult injury that could
become lethal with delayed treatment. The major aspects of
diagnosis and treatment in the primary and secondary surveys
are covered below. At the outset, all trauma patients should be
immobilized with a spinal board and cervical collar and be
given 100% oxygen until they have been fully evaluated and
stabilized.

I. PRIMARY SURVEY

A. AIRWAY

All patients are at risk of airway compromise from vomiting,
and those at significant risk of airway compromise include
patients with maxillofacial injury, burn inhalation injury, and
direct trauma to the neck or larynx. Signs of airway obstruction
include agitation (hypoxia), cyanosis, noisy breathing (snoring,
gurgling, stridor), hoarseness, and palpable deformity or
deviation of trachea. See Chapter 1 for more information about
the airway.

1. Airway Maintenance:

Finger sweep, chin lift or jaw thrust, oropharyngeal or
nasopharyngeal airway

2. Definitive Airway:

Three varieties—orotracheal, nasotracheal, or surgical.
Intubation is indicated for the following:
   a. Apnea
   b. Inability to maintain a patent airway by other means
   c. To protect airway from aspiration of blood or vomit
   d. To prevent airway compromise by inhalation injury,
      maxillofacial trauma, cervical trauma, seizures
   e. Closed head injury requiring assisted ventilation (Glasgow
      Coma Score [GCS] <9)
   f. Inability to maintain oxygenation despite oxygen
      supplementation

3. Decision Making in Airway Management:

a. Assume spinal cord injury in all patients.

b. If breathing, place nasotracheal tube with in-line manual cervical traction by second assistant. Contraindicated with evidence of facial or skull fractures.

c. If apneic or if unable to intubate breathing patient nasotracheally, place orotracheal tube with traction (this may require rapid-sequence intubation with an induction agent and a neuromuscular blocking agent).

d. Surgical airway indicated if unable to perform endotracheal intubation after three attempts. Cricothyroidotomy (not tracheostomy) procedure of choice via vertical skin incision. Jet insufflation via 12- to 14-inch catheter is a temporary alternative if inadequate resources for cricothyroidotomy.

B. BREATHING AND VENTILATION

The chest and neck are exposed to assess breathing and the neck veins.

1. Tension Pneumothorax:

A clinical diagnosis; differentiate from cardiac tamponade. Immediate treatment accomplished with large-bore needle placed in second intercostal space, midclavicular line. Definitively treated by chest tube at fifth intercostal space (nipple level), anterior to midaxillary line.

2. Flail Chest:

Multiple rib fractures. May be hypoxic from underlying pulmonary contusion.

3. Massive Hemothorax:

Requires thoracostomy with 36F chest tube. If >1000 ml drained initially or continued instability, prepare for thoracotomy.

4. Open Pneumothorax (Sucking Chest Wound):

Initial treatment is placement of sterile occlusive dressing taped on three sides to create flutter valve, followed by chest tube placed at a site remote from the wound.

C. CIRCULATION

1. Shock:

Recognize shock; search for and treat its cause. Assume hypovolemic shock from hemorrhage until proven otherwise. Rule out nonhemorrhagic shock states:

a. Cardiogenic (tamponade, myocardial contusion, infarction, air embolus). Perform pericardiocentesis if shock exists in a patient with elevated neck veins without a tension pneumothorax.

b. Neurogenic (spinal cord injury, not intracranial injury).

c. Septic (rare in acute trauma but possible with delayed presentation).

d. Shock caused by tension pneumothorax (because of decreased venous return to the heart).

2. Hemorrhagic Shock Classification:

a. Class I: Blood volume loss <15%. Mild tachycardia usually is the only sign.

b. Class II: Blood volume loss 15%–30%. Signs include tachycardia, tachypnea, decreased pulse pressure, anxiety.

c. Class III: Blood volume loss 30%–40%. Marked tachycardia and tachypnea, significant mental status changes, decreased systolic blood pressure.

d. Class IV: Blood volume loss >40%. Marked tachycardia, hypotension, very narrow pulse pressure, obtundation.

3. Interventions:

a. Control external bleeding with direct pressure if possible.

b. Two large-caliber (16-gauge or larger) peripheral intravenous (IV) lines. May also obtain central access (femoral, jugular, or subclavian vein) or perform saphenous vein cutdown. Consider intraosseous infusion before central line attempt in a child <6 years old.

c. Crystalloid infusion—Ringer's lactate (preferred) or normal saline. Initial bolus is 1–2 l for adult, 20 ml/kg for pediatric patient. Use 3:1 rule: crystalloid needed = 3× blood loss.

d. Type-specific blood or O negative blood for type III and type IV hemorrhagic shock.

e. Send patient's blood for type and cross-match, hemoglobin, chemistries, and B-hCG in female patients.

f. With central access, can use rapid infuser (level I) to deliver large volumes of warmed fluids.

D. DISABILITY

Brief neurological assessment. Level of consciousness may be described by AVPU method (alert, responsive to vocal stimuli, responsive to painful stimuli, unresponsive), but GCS is more detailed and predictive of outcome. Altered mental status may be caused by hypoxia, shock, drugs, or alcohol, but consider it due to traumatic central nervous system injury until proven otherwise. Document focal neurological deficits.

E. EXPOSURE AND ENVIRONMENTAL CONTROL

Refers to physical exposure of the patient by undressing and examining for less obvious signs of trauma, and treatment of or prevention of hypothermia.

1. Undress Patient:
   a. Remove all clothing, jewelry, etc.
   b. Log-roll the patient to examine all surfaces, including ventral and dorsal surfaces, intertriginous areas, perineum.
   c. "Fingers and tubes in every orifice": Examine auditory canals, nose, mouth, rectum, vagina if indicated (rape or perineal trauma).
   d. Never assume a patient with blunt trauma does not have penetrating trauma—always search carefully for stab or puncture wounds, bullet holes.

2. Prevent Hypothermia:
   Cover patient once fully examined with warm blankets or warming device (Bair Hugger); infuse crystalloids via fluid warmer.

II. RESUSCITATION AND ADJUNCTIVE MONITORING

A. MONITOR PATIENT

Continuous electrocardiogram monitoring, pulse oximetry, frequent vital sign checks

B. URINARY CATHETER (FOLEY)

1. Place Urinary Catheter:

   Urine output allows estimate of the patient's volume status.

2. Contraindications:

   a. Urethral damage, especially in male patients, due to longer urethra
   b. Blood at the penile meatus
   c. Blood/ecchymosis of scrotum
   d. High-riding or floating prostate on rectal examination

C. NASOGASTRIC TUBE

Place a nasogastric tube to decompress the stomach; also may prevent emesis and aspiration. Contraindications: maxillofacial trauma. Cribriform plate fracture may allow nasogastric tube to pass into brain. If facial fractures are suspected, use an orogastric tube.

D. RADIOGRAPHS

1. Obtain After Stabilization of Patient:

   Radiographs should be obtained once the patient is stabilized. Do not delay evaluation and resuscitation while waiting for radiographs.

2. Views:

   a. Blunt trauma: cervical spine, anteroposterior (AP) chest and AP pelvis are mandatory.
   b. Penetrating trauma: AP chest and radiographs of trauma site, if applicable.
   c. After resuscitation is complete, comprehensive radiograph series such as lumbosacral spine and extremity films may be obtained. CT scanning may be also performed at this point.

III. SECONDARY SURVEY

The secondary survey begins when the primary survey is completed, resuscitative efforts are established, and the patient is stabilizing. It consists of a head-to-toe examination, a reassessment of vital signs, and a complete neurological examination. A history is taken at this time, either from the patient, the paramedics, or any witnesses.

An AMPLE history of the patient includes allergies, medications, past medical/surgical history, last meal, and exposures (past and present) such as tetanus immunization, alcohol/drugs, etc.

The incident history should be obtained from the patient and paramedics, if possible.

> Blunt trauma: estimate speed of vehicle, vector, damage, steering wheel deformity, status of windshield, fate of other occupants and crash victims, history of ejection, seatbelt usage.
> Penetrating trauma: bullet caliber, distance from shooter, number of shots heard.
> Burns: associated smoke inhalation, explosion, falling objects, chemicals or toxins.
> Cold or heat exposure.

A. HEAD

1. Examination:

Check for external signs of head injury, such as scalp/face lacerations, palpable facial or depressed skull fractures. Perform ophthalmologic examination (pupillary reflexes, extraocular movement, visual acuity if appropriate; rule out foreign body or penetrating injury to globe).

2. Glasgow Coma Score:

a. Assessment of eye opening (1–4)
b. Assessment of verbal response (1–5)
c. Assessment of motor response (1–6)
d. Potential for severe central nervous system (CNS) injury is high if GCS <9, moderate if between 9–12.

3. CT Scan:

Procedure of choice if CNS injury or epidural or subdural hematoma is suspected.

B. MAXILLOFACIAL

Assess for stability, fractures, airway patency. Check for malocclusion or missing teeth.

C. CERVICAL SPINE

If the cervical spine films do not reveal a fracture or dislocation, and the patient is alert and nonintoxicated, the collar may be removed if the patient's clinical exam is normal. Note: if palpation along the cervical spine or range of motion produces pain, replace the collar and obtain full radiologic evaluation of the cervical spine. Often this requires CT scanning, MRI and flexion/extension views of the cervical spine. Cervical spine control is fundamental at all times during airway management.

1. Traction:

If immobilization devices are unavailable, manual in-line traction is necessary.

2. Contraindications:

The cervical spine should be considered unstable (pending radiology) if any of the following are present:
   a. Physical examination reveals a neurological deficit, bony abnormality, or midline tenderness.
   b. The patient has experienced multisystem trauma, a blunt injury above the clavicle, or an altered level of consciousness.
   c. Maxillofacial/head trauma is present.

3. Radiologic Evaluation:

Obtain at least three views of the cervical spine (lateral, odontoid, and AP).

D. NECK

Evaluate for carotid or tracheolaryngeal trauma: carotid bruits, subcutaneous emphysema, expanding hematoma.

E. CHEST

Palpate all ribs, clavicles, and sternum for tenderness; assess symmetrical expansion; auscultate all lung fields and heart sounds (decreased in tamponade). Evaluate chest radiograph for rib fractures, pneumothorax, hemothorax, widened mediastinum.

F. ABDOMEN

Auscultate and palpate all four quadrants; assess penetrating injuries. Reassess frequently because examination may change with time.

1. Investigations:

Patients with unexplained hypotension, neurological injury, impaired sensorium, and equivocal abdominal findings should be considered for peritoneal lavage, abdominal ultrasound (in the trauma bay), or CT scan if the patient is hemodynamically stable. These studies should also be considered if the patient has pelvic or lower rib fractures that prevent accurate assessment of pain, or if the patient is to receive a general anesthetic for other reasons.

    a. Diagnostic peritoneal lavage (DPL) (Chapter 5):
- Allows quick evaluation in trauma bay, with full resuscitation equipment nearby.
- Sensitivity approaches 98% (may miss retroperitoneal injuries).
- Positive if gross blood; >100,000 RBC/hpf; >500 WBC/hpf; or if bile, pancreatic juice, urine, succus, or stool is returned.
- Only absolute contraindication is obvious need for celiotomy.
- Relative contraindications: previous abdominal operations, obesity, cirrhosis, coagulopathy.
- Use supraumbilical incision if pelvic fracture suspected to avoid entering hematoma.

    b. Focused abdominal sonography for trauma (FAST) (see Appendix B)
- Accuracy comparable to DPL and CT in experienced hands.
- Rapid, noninvasive, inexpensive, easily repeatable.
- Obtain a control scan 30 minutes after the first scan to detect slow bleeding.

    c. CT scan
- More fully evaluates retroperitoneal structures and potential pelvic fractures.
- Overall less sensitive but more specific than peritoneal lavage for intraperitoneal injuries.
- Requires transport to scanner, away from full resuscitation equipment.
- Time consuming, requires administration of oral and intravenous contrast.

    d. Contrast studies

Special contrast studies that may be indicated include urethrography, cystography, one-shot intravenous pyelogram (IVP), upper GI series or gastrograffin enema.

2. Absolute Indications for Celiotomy:
   a. Blunt trauma with positive DPL or ultrasound, or recurrent hypotension
   b. Peritonitis
   c. Penetrating trauma with hypotension or bleeding from the stomach, rectum, or genitourinary tract
   d. Gunshot wounds traversing the peritoneal cavity or retroperitoneum
   e. Evisceration

G. PERINEUM
Observe for hematoma; perform pelvic examination in female patients and rectal examination in all patients.

H. MUSCULOSKELETAL SYSTEM
Pelvic rocking may elicit pain in patients with fractures; evaluate all extremities. Missed extremity fractures are quite common, especially if the patient has multisystem trauma. Occasionally, occult pelvic fractures will not be discovered until the patient feels pain when attempting to walk. Attempt to reduce and splint fractures after primary survey, do not attempt to reduce dislocated joints. Beware associated vascular injuries, compartment syndrome, exsanguination with pelvic fractures.

I. SPINAL CORD
Evaluate pupils, cranial nerves, sensation/motor activity in extremities, rectal tone. Treat neurogenic shock, keep immobilized until instability is ruled out, document level and severity of deficit. Beware of loss of respiratory function with high cervical cord injury. Neurosurgical consultation is mandatory if spinal cord injury is suspected. For blunt spinal cord injury, current standard of care in North America includes high-dose steroids within 8 hours of injury: Methylprednisolone, 30 mg/kg loading dose, then 5.4 mg/kg per hour over 23 hours.

IV. SPECIAL CONSIDERATIONS

A. THERMAL INJURIES

B. TRAUMA IN PREGNANCY

C. PEDIATRIC TRAUMA

D. TRAUMA IN ELDERLY OR ATHLETES

REFERENCES

1. Cummins RO (ed): Textbook of Advanced Cardiac Life Support. Dallas, American Heart Association, 1994, pp 1–39.
2. American Heart Association, Emergency Cardiac Care Committee and Subcommittees: Guidelines for cardiopulmonary resuscitation and emergency cardiac care. JAMA 268:2171–2295, 1992.
3. Subcommittee on Advanced Trauma Life Support: Advanced Cardiac Life Support for Doctors, 6th ed. Chicago, American College of Surgeons, 1997, pp 9–324.

APPENDIX B
FOCUSED ABDOMINAL SONOGRAM FOR TRAUMA (FAST)

Author: Jason Lee Sperry, M.D.

Ultrasound has become a useful, noninvasive tool for surgeons to use in gathering diagnostic information to determine whether operative intervention is required in the trauma setting. Studies report a sensitivity of 69% to 98% and a specificity of 95% to 99% when ultrasound is performed by trauma surgeons with appropriate training.

FAST provides a fast noninvasive examination of the dependent regions of the pericardial sac and abdomen for detection of fluid (blood) in the acute trauma setting. This examination can be performed correctly with appropriate training in an average of 2–4 minutes.

1. Indications:

    All trauma patients, after the initial primary survey, who do not already require emergent operative intervention

2. Contraindications:

    None

3. Anesthesia:

    None

4. Equipment:

    a. 3.5-MHz ultrasound probe and monitor
    b. Water-soluble hypoallergenic transmission gel

5. Positioning:

    Supine

6. Technique:

a. After initial stabilization and primary survey, warmed ultrasound gel is applied to four areas in the thoracoabdominal region (see Figure):

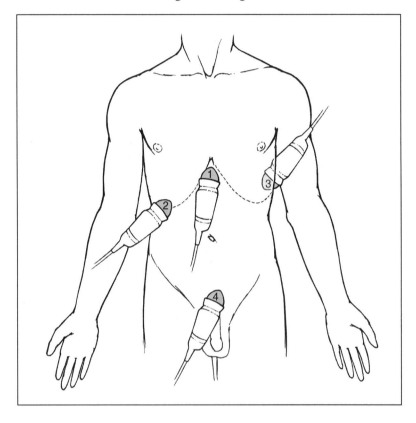

- Pericardial area
- Right upper quadrant
- Left upper quadrant
- Pouch of Douglas (suprapubic area)

b. The transducer is oriented for sagittal sections and then placed first over the subxiphoid region to examine the heart and pericardial sac for blood.

c. The transducer is placed over the right midaxillary line between the eleventh and twelfth ribs.

- Examine the sagittal section of the liver, kidney, and diaphragm
- Examine Morison's pouch for blood

    d. The transducer is placed over the left posterior axillary line between the eleventh and twelfth ribs.
- Examine the spleen and kidney
- Examine the splenorenal recess and subdiaphragmatic space for blood

    e. Lastly, the transducer is placed 4 cm superior to the symphysis pubis, directed for coronal sections, and then moved inferiorly in a side-to-side fashion to examine the bladder and pouch of Douglas for blood.

APPENDIX C
CONSCIOUS IV SEDATION

Author: Christopher J. Sonnenday, M.D.

The performance of certain bedside surgical procedures may lead to significant pain and discomfort for patients. Proper care of a patient undergoing such a procedure requires not only technical skill and preparation in the performance of the procedure, but the provision of adequate anesthesia as well. When surgical procedures take place outside of the operating room or intensive care unit, special precautions must be observed to ensure the safe administration of analgesic and amnestic agents.

Conscious sedation is defined as the achievement of a minimally depressed level of consciousness that retains the patient's ability to maintain a patent airway. Administering safe conscious sedation for patients undergoing a procedure requires knowledge of appropriate medications and adherence to a strict set of guidelines for monitoring of patients during and after sedative use. Sedation protocols are hospital-based; any personnel involved in the administration of sedation and performance of bedside procedures should be familiar with these protocols. Several principles, described below, are essential to any conscious sedation protocol. Each physician should be familiar with the dosing, adverse effects, and expected action of a few sedation agents, as outlined below. Careful attention should be paid to the response of each individual to a particular medication, and sedatives should be slowly titrated to effect rather than administered in large initial doses. In addition, sedation cannot substitute for appropriate topical or local anesthesia.

A. CONSCIOUS SEDATION PROTOCOL

1. Personnel:

Conscious sedation for surgical procedures requires an operator, typically a physician, and a monitor, which may be a registered nurse or another physician. Each of these participants should be trained in advanced cardiac life support (ACLS). Proper support, that is, attending physicians and senior residents, additional nursing staff, and anesthesiologists, should be readily available.

2. Equipment:

Essential equipment includes monitors capable of continuous cardiac monitoring, periodic noninvasive blood pressure measurement, and pulse oximetry. An oxygen source and face mask/cannula should always be used. Other equipment needed at every bedside procedure requiring sedation includes a suction device, bag–mask set-up, oropharyngeal/nasopharyngeal airways, and an emergency box including intubation equipment, a defibrillator, and ACLS medications.

3. Preprocedure Assessment:

Patient information, including allergies, current medications, last oral intake, difficult airway/anesthesia experiences, and pregnancy, should be reviewed by the personnel involved in the procedure. Particular attention should be paid to patients with risk factors for aspiration, including obesity, pregnancy, gastroesophageal reflux disease, diabetes mellitus, and head trauma, and patients with an altered level of consciousness. More invasive and skilled monitoring, particularly with the presence of an anesthesiologist, should be considered in these high-risk patients. Preprocedure vital signs and assessment, including baseline level of consciousness, should be recorded prior to any intervention. Establishment of a reliable, patent intravenous access at this time is essential.

4. Monitoring:

Assessment of mental status, airway protection, and vital signs should be made on a minute-to-minute basis, following hospital protocols. In the event of loss of airway protection, absence of responsiveness, or oxygen desaturation, the procedure should be suspended. The patient should be stimulated, and the airway protected with a jaw thrust, chin lift, and/or oral airway (see Chapter 1). Mechanical bag–mask ventilation may be initiated. Reversal agents should be considered, and anesthesia assistance should be called as soon as concern about the patency of the patient's airway is noted. In the event of the need for resuscitation, ACLS protocols should be followed.

5. Discharge Criteria:

Monitoring of the patient should continue until the patient meets established post-procedure discharge criteria. This includes return to baseline mobility; return to an awake, oriented or baseline mental status; stable vital signs; and demonstration of the ability to safely protect the airway—adequate cough, gag, and ability to take oral intake.

B. SYSTEMIC ANALGESICS

1. Morphine:

Reliable opioid that is carefully titrated to clinical effect while the patient is closely monitored for respiratory depression.
  a. Initial dose: 1–2 mg titrated every 5–15 minutes
  b. Expected total dose: 0.1 mg/kg
  c. Onset: 1–3 minutes
  d. Duration: 3–5 hours
  e. Side effects: Hypotension, respiratory depression, bronchospasm, urinary retention, constipation, pruritus. Synergistic effects when combined with benzodiazepines.

2. Fentanyl:

An alternative to morphine preferred in many cases because of its quicker onset and shorter duration of action. Fentanyl also tends to cause less histamine release in comparison with morphine, thus limiting, but not removing, the risk of pruritus and bronchospasm.
  a. Initial dose: 25–50 µg IV titrated every 4–6 minutes
  b. Expected total dose: 1–3 µg/kg
  c. Onset: 30–120 seconds
  d. Duration: 30–60 minutes
  e. Side effects/comments: As above for morphine

3. Meperidine:

An alternative in patients with allergies to other agents. Usually not preferred due to its ability to cause seizures at high doses or in patients with inhibited clearance.
  a. Initial dose: 25–50 mg titrated every 5–10 minutes
  b. Expected total dose: 1–2 mg/kg
  c. Onset: 1–2 minutes
  d. Duration: 2–4 hours

e. Side effects: As above for morphine. Additionally, meperidine may have catastrophic interactions with monamine oxidase inhibitors. Toxic metabolite, normeperidine, may cause seizures.

C. SEDATION/AMNESTIC AGENTS

1. Midazolam:

Rapid-acting benzodiazepine that is easily and safely titrated to clinical effect.
   a. Initial dose: 0.5–1.0 mg titrated every 4–5 minutes
   b. Expected total dose: 0.05–0.1 mg/kg
   c. Onset: 1 minute
   d. Duration: 1–2 hours
   e. Side effects: Potentiates respiratory depression and hypotension in combination with narcotics. May cause paradoxical disinhibition, especially in elderly patients.

2. Diazepam:

Longer acting benzodiazepine.
   a. Initial dose: 1–2 mg titrated every 6–10 minutes
   b. Expected total dose: 0.1 mg/kg
   c. Onset: 1–5 minutes
   d. Duration: 1–4 hours
   e. Side effects: As above for midazolam. May cause phlebitis upon injection.

3. Droperidol:

Sedative with antiemetic effects that may markedly enhance the effects of narcotics and other sedatives.
   a. Initial dose: 1.25–2.5 mg titrated every 5–7 minutes
   b. Expected total dose: Maximal dose 6.25 mg
   c. Onset: 3–10 minutes
   d. Duration: 2–4 hours
   e. Side effects: Similar to midazolam. May have powerful sedative effects, especially in the elderly, or with concomitant narcotic administration.

D. REVERSAL AGENTS

1. Flumazenil:

   Benzodiazepine antagonist.
   a. Dose: 0.2 mg every minute up to 1.0 mg
   b. Expected total dose: Maximal dose 1.0 mg
   c. Onset: 30–60 seconds
   d. Duration: 45–90 minutes
   e. Side effects: May precipitate excessive catecholamine state
      secondary to reversal of sedation; may cause seizures in
      patients with history of benzodiazepine abuse. Sedation
      may recur secondary to short half-life of flumazenil relative
      to benzodiazepines. A continuous infusion of 0.5–1.0
      µg/kg/min may be necessary until the benzodiazepine is
      fully metabolized.

2. Naloxone:

   Opioid receptor antagonist.
   a. Initial dose: 0.1–0.2 mg every 2–3 minutes
   b. Expected total dose: 0.1 mg/kg
   c. Onset: 1–5 minutes
   d. Duration: 30–60 minutes
   e. Side effects: May precipitate excessive catecholamine state
      secondary to reversal of sedation. Sedation may recur
      secondary to short half-life of naloxone. Continuous
      infusion of 5–40 µg/h may be necessary until the narcotic
      has been fully metabolized.

APPENDIX D
SUTURE BASICS

Jon D. Vogel, M.D.

Tensile Strength: The weight required to break a suture ÷ The cross-sectional area of the suture. Decreased cross-sectional area → increased number of zeroes in the suture size (4-0 vs. 2-0) → decreased tensile strength.

Tissue Reactivity: Natural fibers (silk and gut) cause more inflammation than synthetic fibers, like PDS and Vicryl.

Configuration: Twisted, braided, or monofilament.

Knot Security: Braided and uncoated sutures hold the knot better.

Infection Risk: Braided suture can harbor bacteria, which increases the risk of infection.

Absorbable Sutures

Suture	Trade Names	Configuration	Tensile Strength Loss (days)*	Tissue Reaction	Common Uses
Fast gut		Twisted	3–5	++++	Scalp and facial lacerations in children
Plain gut		Twisted	5–7	++++	Vessel ligation, mucosa
Chromic gut		Twisted	10–14	+++	Vessel ligation, mucosa, GI tract, viscera
Polyglecaprone 25	Monocryl†	Monofilament	7	+	Subcutaneous tissue, skin, GI tract
Polyglycolic acid	Dexon†	Braided	14–21	++	GI tract, vessel ligation
Polygalactic acid	Vicryl§	Braided	14–21	++	Fascia, viscera, GI tract, muscle, vessel ligation
Polydioxanone	PDS§	Monofilament	28	+	Fascia, cosmetic closures, GI tract, muscle
Polyglyconate	Maxon†	Monofilament	28	+	GI tract, cosmetic closures, muscle, fascia

*Time to 50% strength loss.
†Trade names are of the Ethicon company.
§Trade names are of the Davis & Geck company.

Nonabsorbable Sutures

Suture	Trade Names	Configuration	Tensile Strength	Tissue Reaction	Common Uses
Silk	Perma-Hand*	Braided	Good	++++	Vessel ligation, GI tract
Nylon	Ethilon* Dermalon†	Monofilament	High	+	Skin, drain stitches, fascia, vasculature
Nylon	Nurolon* Surgilon†	Braided	High	++	Neurosurgery, tendons
Polypropylene	Prolene* Surgilene†	Monofilament	Good	+	Cardiac tissue, vasculature, fascia, skin, tendons, neurosurgery
Polyester	Ethibond* Tycron†	Braided	High	++	Cardiac tissue, vascular, fascia, tendon
Polybutester	Novofil*	Monofilament	High	++	Fascia, ligaments, tendons
Stainless steel	Ethisteel* Flexon†	Monofilament	High	+	Sternal closure, orthopedics, drain stitches, fascia

*Trade names are of the Davis & Geck company.
†Trade names are of the Ethicon company.

Suture Needles

Needle Types	Description	Pros and Cons	Common Uses
Conventional cutting _PS-1, 3, 5* _SCE-2†	Three cutting edges including concavity ▲ Tapers to sharp point	Ease of tissue penetration High risk of cut-out	Cosmetic surgery, sternal closure
Reverse cutting _P1, FS1, OS-8, KS (Keith)* _CE-4, 6, 8†	Three cutting edges including convexity ▶ Tapers to sharp point	Ease of tissue penetration Lower risk of cut-out KS: Needle holder not required	Skin, tendons, fascia, cosmetic surgery, ENT
Taper point _RB1, SH1, CTX* _T-8, T-19†	No cutting edges • Tapers to sharp point	Small needle hole ↓ leak around suture	Biliary tree, dura, fascia, GI tract, muscle, peritoneum, pleura, subcutaneous fat
Reverse cut/taper _CC, V4* _DTE-1, DT-5†	Body of needle tapers into a reverse-cutting ▶ sharp tip •	Taper point gives benefit of easier tissue penetration	Calcified tissue, fascia, ligaments
Blunt point _CTX-B, BP* _MT-56†	Tapered needle body • with blunt point	Decreased tissue tearing and bleeding	Visceral organs, fascia, GI tract

▲ = Needle tip concavity; ▼ = needle tip convexity; • = needle tip sharply pointed.
*Trade names are of the Davis & Geck company.
†Trade names are of the Ethicon company.

INDEX

References in *italics* indicate figures